Black, White or Mixed Race?

The number of people in racially mixed relationships has grown steadily over the last thirty years, yet many people still stigmatise them and expect them to feel unhappy about their identities.

The first edition of *Black, White or Mixed Race?* was a ground-breaking study; this revised edition uses new literature to consider what is now known about racialised identities, changes in the official use of 'mixed' categories and the implications for transracial adoption. These new developments are placed in a historical framework and in the context of up-to-date literature on mixed parentage in Britain and the USA.

Based on research with young people from a range of social back-grounds the book examines their attitudes to black and white people; their identity; their cultural origins; their friendships; their experiences of racism. This was the first British study to concentrate on adolescents of black and white parentage and it continues to provide unique insights into their identities. It is a valuable resource for all those concerned with social work and policy and for researchers in psychology and the social sciences.

Barbara Tizard is Emeritus Professor at the Institute of Education, London. **Ann Phoenix** is Senior Lecturer in Psychology at The Open University.

Black, White or Mixed Race?

Race and racism in the lives of
young people of mixed parentage

Revised Edition

Barbara Tizard and Ann Phoenix

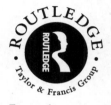

London and New York

First edition published 1993; this revised edition published 2002
by Routledge
11 New Fetter Lane, London EC4P 4EE

Simultaneously published in the USA and Canada
by Routledge
29 West 35th Street, New York, NY 10001

Routledge is an imprint of the Taylor & Francis Group

© 2002 Barbara Tizard and Ann Phoenix

Typeset in Times by RefineCatch Limited, Bungay, Suffolk
Printed and bound in Great Britain by
TJ International Ltd, Padstow, Cornwall

British Library Cataloguing in Publication Data
A catalogue record for this book is available from the British Library

Library of Congress Cataloging in Publication Data
Tizard, Barbara.
    Black, white or mixed race?: race and racism in the lives of young
people of mixed parentage/Barbara Tizard and Ann Phoenix.—Rev.
ed.
        p. cm.
    Includes bibliographical references and index.
    1. Racially mixed children. I Phoenix, Ann. II. Title.
HQ777.9.T59 2001
306.84′6—dc21
                                                    2001041846

ISBN 0–415–25981–9 (hbk.)
ISBN 0–415–25982–7 (pbk.)

Printed and bound by Antony Rowe Ltd, Eastbourne

Contents

vi *Contents*

Acknowledgements

The research discussed in this book was carried out with a grant from the Department of Health. We would particularly like to thank Dr Carolyn Davies, of the Department's Research Management Division, for her support.

We are very grateful to the teachers in the schools where we worked for their co-operation, and in particular to the young people and their parents who enabled us to carry out the research. Les Back, Ann Brackenridge and Wendy Francis were Research Officers on the project. We would like to thank Hilary Chambers, Philip Graham, Peter Honig, Sonia Jackson, Anne Peters and Lucy and Jenny Tizard, who read and commented on part or all of the manuscript, as did Les Back and Ann Brackenridge. Olwen Davies' efficient secretarial service was invaluable throughout the project. Charlie Owen generously helped and advised with computing, and discussed the research with us at all stages. For the first edition he allowed us to refer to his as yet unpublished analysis of recent Labour Force Survey Data, and for this new edition he has continued to provide references, comments and technical support.

1 Setting the scene

Introduction

One of the most striking social trends in Britain is the increasing number of 'interracial' marriages and cohabitations and people of mixed parentage. Despite this trend, 'mixed marriages' are still unusual in Britain. They currently make up just over 1 per cent of all marriages (Berrington, 1996; Owen, 2001). This small overall percentage is not surprising since more than 94 per cent of the British population is white. However, an increasing number of the cohabiting relationships of people of Caribbean origin are with white British people (see Chapter 2).

Recent analyses indicate that there continue to be gender differences in patterns of mixed relationships. Half of British-born men of Caribbean origin who are married or cohabiting are living with a white woman. The comparable proportion of British-born women of Caribbean origin who live with a white man is one-third. Moreover, the rate of mixed partnerships is increasing more rapidly for men of African Caribbean origin than for women (Berthoud, 2001). As we shall document, surveys of white people indicate that their attitudes to interracial unions are more sympathetic today than they were in the past. Much less is known about black attitudes, although there is evidence that black people are more likely than white people to approve of interracial unions. Yet people continue to worry about the children of these unions. Rather than being seen as the fortunate inheritors of two cultures as the children of an Anglo-French marriage might be seen, they are only too often considered objects of pity. One of the authors of this book, when discussing its contents with journalists, met with incredulity when she told them that many young people of mixed parentage see advantages in their situation. Such a view runs counter to the widespread belief that they can be expected to suffer from identity problems, low self-esteem, and problem or delinquent behaviour.

Origins of distaste for racial mixing

The origins of this belief lie deep in theories about 'race' which, while rejected by most contemporary scientists, still maintain their hold on the general public, and form the basis of racism. According to these theories, human beings are divided into distinct biological groups according to skin colour, each with its distinct physical and psychological characteristics. Not surprisingly, since the originators of these theories were white, the white 'race' was said to be superior to all others in intellectual achievement and morality, and the black 'race' inferior, with other 'races' coming in between.

It is, of course, the case that people in different parts of the world tend to have different skin colours, although even in this respect there is overlap – some white people have darker or more sallow skins than some African Caribbean or Asian people. But the idea that different skin colours are associated with different psychological characteristics has long been discredited. Moreover, we know from modern genetics that human beings are not divided into distinct biological 'races'. If they were, the 'races' would have to be distinct from one another in a large number of their genes, not just the genes for skin colour. Yet when genes have been mapped across the world it has been found that trends in skin colour are not accompanied by trends in other genes. Far from it: around 85 per cent of genetic diversity comes from the differences between individuals of the same colour in the same country, for example, two randomly chosen white English people. Another 5–10 per cent comes from differences between people in different countries, for example, England and France. The genetic difference between 'races', for example, Europeans and Africans, is about the same size as the genetic difference between people from different European countries. Human beings, the geneticist Steve Jones (1991) concludes, are a remarkably homogenous species. Biologically, we are all of us multiracial.

Racial classification, with its assertion of the innate superiority of the white 'race', conveniently justified slavery and, later, imperial conquest. To maintain the superiority of the white 'race' it was important to keep it 'pure'. Hence the opposition to, and often outrage at, the idea of marriage between white people and those of other 'races'. It was feared their offspring would not only dilute 'white blood', but that they would disgrace the family by inheriting and transmitting the bad qualities of the inferior 'race', including their stigmatised appearance. Moreover, because of the emphasis on strict racial demarcation, 'mixed-bloods' were seen as anomalies, demonstrably neither one 'race' nor another, and as such they tended to arouse discomfort. Yet paradoxically these despised mixes were created by the sexual activity of white men in the course of enslaving or conquering other peoples.

The distaste for racial mixing was reflected in the names given by white people to those of mixed parentage, which have always had offensive connotations of animal breeding. 'Mulatto', the Portuguese word for a young mule, was in use in the United States and the West Indies from the sixteenth to the twentieth century; 'métis', meaning a mongrel dog, was the French equivalent; 'mixed-breed', and 'half-breed' were used in Britain and the USA; while in the twentieth century 'half-caste' became the commonest term. It was only in countries where people of obvious mixed origin came to form the majority of the population, as in Brazil, that mixed parentage ceased to be a matter for opprobrium.

In the rest of the world they were stigmatised by white people, and often envied and distrusted by black or Asian people for the preferential treatment they might receive. In some countries they were numerous enough to form a viable community, run their own schools and newspapers, and have their own politicians and poets. This was the case, for example, with Anglo-Indians in India, Eurasians in Indonesia and coloureds in Guyana (Gist and Dworkin, 1972). There, despite rejection from other groups, they must have gained strength from a sense of community identity. In the USA, although people of mixed parentage were quite numerous in some parts, the 'one drop of black blood' rule adopted after the abolition of slavery meant they were classified as black. Most of them probably internalised this rule and assumed a black identity, while a few 'passed' as white. But by the 1950s more than one third were said to identify with both black and white people (Spickard, 1989: 333).

In Britain there were no legal definitions of a black person, or legal restrictions on mixed marriages. This may have been in part because until the mid-1950s the number of black people in Britain was very small – never more than 15,000, often less. The few 'half-castes' were generally recognised by both black and white people as different from black. But they were stigmatised as much in Britain as elsewhere, perhaps more so, since they were usually born into the poorest sector of society, while in other countries they tended to be part of an intermediate class.

Signs of change

Since the 1960s there have been major changes in both Britain and the USA that seem likely to have led to both black and mixed-parentage people developing more positive identities. The scientific discrediting of theories about the superiority of the white 'race', and the increasing liberalisation of white attitudes, have tended to reduce the stigma attached to being black or of mixed parentage. The success of the black consciousness movement in raising black self-esteem has probably had an even more important effect, both on the identity of black people and on white attitudes to them. But paradoxically, the rise of the black consciousness movement led to a renewed insistence on the 'one drop of black blood makes a person black' rule, this time on the part of black people. They argued strongly that pride in being a person of colour should lead people of mixed parentage to regard themselves, and be regarded by others, as black. Any other identity was seen as a betrayal, a rejection of their black ancestry.

Although in Britain this view was accepted by white social workers, social scientists and people in the media, it is not at all clear to what extent it was accepted among the general public, both black and white, and among mixed-parentage people themselves. The findings we report in this book helped to bring to public consciousness the information that a sizeable proportion of young people reject, or are unaware of, the view. In the USA it was much more widely accepted that people of mixed parentage should be considered black, but in the closing decade of the twentieth century this began to be questioned. People of mixed parentage argued that to deny the white part of their inheritance is psychologically damaging, and in effect involves accepting the discredited racial theory that everyone belongs to one of three or four distinct 'races'. In their view individuals should be able to claim simultaneous membership of whichever groups they choose to identify with. This change in attitude followed the recent expansion of the mixed-parentage population in the USA, especially of people of mixed Japanese and white origin. By the end of the twentieth century, there were estimated to be a million 'biracial' children and adolescents in the USA (Gibbs and Hines, 1992: 223). At least thirty different organisations had been set up with the aim of helping 'biracial' or 'multiracial' people – both terms are used – to affirm both their heritages.

The number of people of mixed parentage has also increased in Britain, and, as we shall show, it is likely that many of them have opted for a dual identity. In Britain there are now organisations particularly for those of 'mixed parentage' as well as for those in 'mixed relationships'.

Even officialdom has begun to recognise this identity. This is demonstrated in the changes in the question on ethnic group between the 1991 and 2001 British, and the 1990 and 2000 US Censuses. The 1991 Census, the first to include a question on ethnic group, offered a curious mixture of racial and national categories, but did not invite or encourage a declaration of mixed origins. People were asked to state to which of the following groups they considered they belonged: 'White, Black-Caribbean, Black-African, Black-Other (please describe), Indian, Pakistani, Bangladeshi, Chinese, Any other ethnic group (please describe).' Only one choice was allowed. There was no invitation to describe oneself as of mixed origin, an affiliation which could only be included in the 'Black-Other' or 'Other' categories. In the British Census of 2001, people who wanted to tick a 'mixed' box could choose from 'White and Black Caribbean'; 'White and Black African'; 'White and Asian'; 'Any other Mixed background, please write in'. While this wording has been criticised for not allowing people of 'mixed ethnic background' to be recognised as British (unlike white, Asian and black groups, but like Chinese groups), it marks an important shift in thinking about 'race' and ethnicity in Britain. This shift is also evident in the USA where, despite a long history of enumerating ethnicity, people of mixed parentage were, for the first time, included as a separate ethnic group in the 2000 Census. Seven million (2.4 per cent) of the US population chose to take up this option (*The Economist*, 2001).

Why such rapid change?

How can we account for such rapid social changes? We would suggest that two sets of conceptual changes have intersected to produce a flourishing of interest in 'mixed parentage' and new ways of thinking about it. First, there has been an expansion of interest in identities and how we think about them. In a nutshell, those changes are such that it is generally accepted that people have several identities at the same time (Hall, 1996). The construction of 'mixed parentage' as necessarily problematic has occurred, and continues to occur, in a context where it is taken for granted as common sense that there are clearly differentiated 'races' who are, in essence, binary opposites. This 'essentialism' has been much criticised in feminist, cultural studies and social science literature because it treats people as though they possess characteristics which are unchanging and which, for example, unite them with those within their 'race' and necessarily differentiate them from those outside the 'race' (Brah, 1996). Such bipolar constructions of black people and white people have been responsible for notions that people can be 'between two cultures' or 'neither one colour nor the other' and denials that it is possible to have identities which are 'both/and', rather than 'either/or' (Collins, 1990).

The idea that we all have multiple identities has also had an impact on thinking about 'race'. Many academics who research and write on 'race' now argue that we can no longer think of black people and white people as opposites or of racism as a single process (Rattansi and Phoenix, 1998). Instead, they suggest that racisms are plural and that what 'race' means and how it is understood changes over time. Both racisms and 'race' are therefore dynamic social processes that are different in different social contexts and for different groups (Brah, 1996). For that reason, many now use the term 'racialisation' which was first coined by the black Martiniquan psychiatrist Frantz Fanon in 1967 to refer to the problems experienced by people who had been colonised (e.g. Banton, 1977; Miles, 1989; Omi and Winant, 1986). Basically, 'racialisation' includes the idea that 'racial meanings' are neither naturally arising nor static but are socially constructed and dynamic social processes. People are therefore 'racialised', rather than having a biological 'race'.

Secondly, since the first edition of this book was published (in 1993) it has become more accepted that people of mixed parentage should be identified separately from the groups to which their parents belong. This is for three reasons:

1   It has become clear that, although there continue to be disputes over terminology, many people of 'mixed parentage' now choose to identify themselves in ways which denote that they have parents who come from groups that are racialised in different ways (e.g. Fatimilehin, 1999). This was one of the main contributions of the first edition of this book.

2   Increasing recognition of 'mixed parentage' in both Britain and the USA has partly resulted from an increase in the number of those in 'mixed relationships' and who are of 'mixed parentage' (Owen, 2001; Phoenix and Owen, 1996/2000).

3   These demographic changes have also served to expand research, autobiographical and popular interest in 'mixed parentage' and 'mixed relationships' both by those who define themselves as 'mixed' and by others (Alibhai-Brown, 2001; Ifekwunigwe, 1999; Katz, 1996; McBride, 1998; Twine, 1999a). Work is beginning to be done on white–Asian mixed parentage (Grove, 1991; Khan, in preparation; Saenz *et al.*, 1995) as well as on white–black mixed parentage.

Understandings of processes of racialisation have intersected with theorisations of 'mixed parentage' to produce richer understandings. Yet, while there has apparently been a progressive recognition of 'mixed parentage', those of 'mixed parentage' and in 'mixed relationships' continue to be subjected to racialised discrimination and disapproval. These contradictions have helped to produce a great deal of resistance to the acceptance of 'mixed parentage' as a conceptual category.

Disputes about terminology

One of the issues faced by those thinking about 'race' and racism is that there are many ways in which the terms 'race', 'racism' and 'ethnicity' are used and disagreements about how they should be used. Furthermore, definitions have tended to shift over time as the boundaries between people constructed as being from different 'races' or ethnic groups have moved. Changes in the meaning and usage of the term 'black' are a case in point. This changed from a term of contempt to the one claimed as the preferred term by black people themselves. The black US scholar Henry Louis Gates (1994: 201) demonstrated this succinctly for a US context: 'The "Personal Statement" for my Yale application began: "My grandfather was colored, my father was Negro, and I am black."' In Britain, the term 'black' has changed from excluding, to including and then excluding again people of Asian descent. Whether or not people of mixed parentage are considered black is a point of contention in discussions of transracial adoption. Shifts have occurred because definitions are a site of dispute not only over what groups should be called, but also over who has the right to define them and who should be included within particular terms.

In Britain and the USA, the conceptual polarisation of black people and white people has, historically, generally led to those of 'mixed parentage' being included in the category now commonly called 'black'. It is indicative of the political nature of this categorisation that having one white parent has never been sufficient to permit inclusion as 'white', but having one black parent necessarily entailed classification as 'black'. Most states (at one time forty of fifty) in the USA enacted laws against 'racially mixed' unions and marriages. Although the categories forbidden to marry in the various states were not consistent, all forbade marriage between black and white people. Such laws were not declared unconstitutional until 1967 (Young, 1995). Definitions of what constituted being black also varied, but, 'in practice – both legal and customary – anyone with *any* known African ancestry was deemed an African American, while only those without any trace of known African ancestry were called Whites' (Spickard, 1992:16). This is what became known as the 'one drop rule' or 'hypodescent'. Common sense would suggest that skin colour was the basis of the black–white differentiation, but as is the case for black people, some people of mixed parentage could be lighter in skin shade than some white people, but would still be classified as black (Spickard, 1992).

The binary thinking (in terms of black people and white people being opposites) that underpinned the 'one drop rule' is still common. For example, arguments that people of mixed parentage have to recognise that, regardless of how they feel, they are black are based on an awareness that racism will differentiate them from white people. Yet, as we have seen above, such arguments construct black people and white people as cultural and visual opposites rather than either as part of a continuum or as connected and/or differentiated by features other than 'race'. Instead of posing a challenge to racism or racialised discourses they (re)produce the 'one drop argument'. Such arguments were commonly rehearsed in the USA as preparations for the 2000 Census were made. The following quotation from the US black magazine *Ebony* illustrates this.

> Some biracial brothers and sisters might do well to heed advice from Lenny Kravitz [American rock star]. 'You don't have to deny the White side of you if you're mixed,' he says. 'Accept the blessing of having the advantage of two cultures, but understand that you are Black. In this world, if you have one spot of Black blood, you are *Black*. So get over it.'
>
> (Norment, 1995: 112)

The fact that the title of the *Ebony* magazine article was: 'Am I black, white or in between? Is there a plot to create a "colored" buffer race in America?' captures longstanding concerns on the part of black people that people of 'mixed parentage' are likely to be 'race traitors' (Root, 1996). Jones (1994) similarly argues that calls to be recognised as 'biracial' dilute black struggle and are misplaced. While he recognises that they arise from pain and resentment at being forced to consider themselves black, he says:

> African Americans have achieved so much in the battle against race as *Black people* that most are little minded to put aside blackness, on the grounds that if Whites recognize some Blacks as bi-racial this will undercut racism. Most Blacks have no intention of claiming a special bi-racial status for themselves while leaving behind

those Blacks who can make no such claim. Bi-racials who mislike this reality may, of course, and should continue their appeals to Whites for special recognition. Those who understand it should rejoin the African American community and continue the struggle for racial justice. There will be time enough to talk about being bi-racial and multi-racial when that struggle is won and Whites are no longer regarded as superior to Blacks.

(Jones, 1994: 209).

Although people with one black and one white parent have historically been categorised as black, they have, simultaneously (and contradictor-ily) been identified as separate from both black and white people. The chromatism or colourism on which 'pigmentocracy' operated inflects colonial history (and, to some extent, still operates). 'Elaborate distinc-tions were made between people on the basis of their racial ancestry and physical attributes. This placed the pure white at the apex of a complex listing of the races and the pure African at the bottom' (Mama, 1995: 102). Paradoxically, while people of mixed parentage (black-white and 'Anglo-Indian') gained privileges on the basis of being closer to whiteness than black people, they were also much des-pised by whites since they symbolised loss of purity of the white 'race'. Young (1995: 180) suggests that 'none was so demonised as those of mixed "race"'.

People of mixed parentage have thus long been positioned in contra-dictory ways – as black and as different from black as well as white people. The specific terms commonly used to describe people of mixed parentage and sexual unions between black and white people tend to pathologise those who cannot easily be fitted into the taken-for-granted racialised binary opposition. Thus 'half-caste', 'mixed race', 'biracial', 'maroon', 'mulatto' and 'métis(se)' all demonstrate essentialism and bipolar thinking. Many are also riven with notions of impurity and references to non-human animals (Root, 1996). In the same way, the terms 'mixed marriage', 'intermarriage' and 'miscegenation' (meaning 'interbreeding between races, especially sexual union of whites with Negroes', *The Shorter Oxford English Dictionary*, 1983) accept binary notions of 'race' and have negative overtones. Perhaps in recognition of the unacceptable overtones of such words, *The Encarta World English Dictionary* (1999) defines miscegenation as a term originating in the mid-nineteenth century that is 'offensive when used disapprovingly, as often formerly'.

Given that there are an increasing number of people who are of mixed parentage and who are in mixed relationships, it is not surprising that this is an area where terminology has been contested. Although this contestation is perhaps less well known than was the contestation over changing the term 'coloured' to 'black' in the 1960s and 1970s, many people now reject usage of terms such as 'mulatto', 'half-caste' and 'miscegenation'. In the USA, where 'Afro-American' has largely given way to African American, there is now widespread usage of the term 'biracial' to make general reference to 'mixed parentage'. In Britain, Small (1986) argued for dropping the term 'mixed race' because it both accepts that there are 'races' and is offensive in denying that children with one black and one white parent are black and will be treated as black by society. He advocated use of the term 'mixed parentage' if 'black' would not suffice. It is true that 'mixed parentage' is, as Small argues, an improvement over 'mixed race' in that it does not explicitly reproduce a binary racialisation. However, although Small does not acknowledge this, it does reproduce racialisation since it is clear that it is not, for example, a mixing of gender that is being evoked. In addition, 'mixed parentage' is unsatisfactory in permanently defining people by the characteristics of their parents.

A further reason for dissatisfaction with the term 'mixed parentage' to describe those who have one black and one white parent is that it constructs an arbitrary division between those of mixed parentage and others. Because the populations of the world are almost all intermixed, most people have some mixed parentage (Small, 1986). Indeed, because of slavery and colonial relationships, many more people are of mixed black-white ancestry than is generally accepted. It is difficult to estimate the percentage of white British and US populations who have black ancestry, but it has been estimated that 70–80 per cent of all US black people have some white ancestry (Zack, 1993). The use of the term 'mixed parentage' is therefore imperfect and provisional, rather than definitive.

Consciousness raising without political organisation

In recent years, there have been attempts to produce terms relating to 'mixed parentage' which are not rooted in the problems discussed above. For example, 'dual heritage' or 'mixed heritage' are gaining popularity as terms which are apparently deracialised and positive, emphasising shared cultural inheritance. The notion of 'dual (or mixed) heritage' is, however, as much a binary construction as is 'half-caste' or 'biracial'. It suggests that we inherit one (or more) culture(s) from each of our birth parents. But culture is complex, intermixed and not genetically inherited. In addition, the notion of heritage reinforces the notion that culture is biologically/genetically produced and transmitted, and suggests that inheritance 'naturally' gives rights to belonging in cultures and nations. This appears inclusive, but reproduces already common exclusions in its implication that belonging is a birthright – something which is not avoided in the innovative 'jewel heritage' used by one of Iyabo Fatimilehin's (1999) research participants. (However, since the participant crossed out this term and substituted 'dual heritage', it is not clear if this was not a phonological error whereby a word pronounced as a homophone was initially recorded.)

A rather different term is favoured by Jayne Ifekwunigwe (1997), who argues for the reclamation of the French term métis(se) and says: 'The English translation . . . is "half caste", "half-breed", or "mongrel". However, it has been re-appropriated by others including myself.' This reappropriation, however, is not akin to the reclamation of the term 'black' in the 1960s and 1970s since that resulted from a popular political movement. For while there are increasing numbers of organisations formed, and conferences held, where people of 'mixed parentage' have been able to meet, these have resulted in crucial consciousness raising, but have not produced clear political strategies or views. This is unlike black political movements which argued for changes in nomenclature as the result of campaigns for wider social changes. The reappropriation of métis(se) may be more akin to the common use of 'nigger' by black rappers – a usage that is less straightforward (Weekes, 1997). However, racialised terms are sometimes successfully reappropriated. For example, the Spanish term 'mestiza(o)' has been reinterpreted by various people in the USA, and the term 'LatiNegra' has been coined for those with African and Latina(o) parentage (Root, 1996).

The term 'black with one white parent' is gaining some popularity on both sides of the Atlantic (Goldstein, 1999; Twine, 1999b) and the term 'black mixed parentage' has also begun to be used (e.g. Banks, 1995). These terms maintain solidarity with black people and potentially give recognition to racisms as affecting people of 'mixed parentage' and 'black' people in similar ways while recognising that some issues are particular to people of mixed parentage. It thus addresses some of the political problems that result from dropping the term 'black' to signify people of 'mixed parentage' without denying the white parent. It can be seen as reproducing essentialist, binary thinking about 'black' and 'white' and so implicitly buttressing old arguments of 'hypodescent' and as challenging such binaries by asserting claims to blackness for those with one white parent. It does make a division between those who are 'Asian with a white parent' and those who are 'black with one white parent'. This may, however, not be problematic in that separate terms now represent 'black people' and 'Asian people'.

The importance of terminological dispute

It is partly because terminology is ideologically marked that some people, particularly those from the white ethnic majority, are diffident about discussing 'race' and racism in case they 'say the wrong thing'. Nonetheless, there are useful ways in which to discuss 'race' and ethnicity while being sensitive to the reasons why terminology remains contested, and hence dynamic. The terms 'race' and 'ethnicity' are all about processes of boundary maintenance in that they are ways of separating 'them' and 'us'. They are thus about social relations, and often help to make constructed, racialised boundaries seem natural.

However unsatisfactory currently used terms may be, the process of questioning meanings is crucial to shifting thinking about mixed parentage. The accounts of the young people of mixed parentage and of people involved in 'racially mixed' relationships presented in this book may be said to demonstrate such a shift. Most of their discourses were not pathological constructions of 'miscegenation' and binary oppositions of 'neither one colour nor the other'. They did, however, use 'half-caste'; 'mixed race' and, in one case, 'métisse' (because the young woman who used it believed it sounded more exotic than English terms). Banks (1999) argues that outsiders to 'mixed parentage' cannot impose terminology on those who are insiders. It may be that, in the future, people who themselves are of mixed parentage will advocate the use of specific terms as a result of political processes similar to those which led to the reclamation of the term 'black' in the 1960s and 1970s. Whatever happens, terminological disputes are always important to the shifting of social constructions and, as such, are often productive. However, since social constructions are dynamic, preferred terms are likely to shift over time:

> There are no terms that are 'right' forever more. Groups define and redefine themselves their sense of who they are culturally and polit-ically as preferred terms change. Also within a group one person may like a term which another may not. We have to constantly pay attention to changing definitions and to the reasons why they are changed. People need to discover for themselves who they are and not have terms imposed on them.
> (Early Years Trainers Anti-Racist Network (EYTARN), 1995: 11)

The terms used in this book

The reader will note that despite condemning the discredited concept of 'race', we continue to use the term ourselves. Others, including official-dom, now prefer the term 'ethnic group'. But an ethnic group refers to people who are constructed as sharing a common history, language, religion and culture. They will usually also have the same skin colour, but people with the same skin colour do not always share a common culture. As we will show, many young British-born people of African Caribbean origin, especially those from middle-class families, have a variety of cultural practices. What sets them apart from white people, and is the basis for their stigmatisation by racists, is their appearance or knowledge that they are of 'mixed parentage', not their culture. It is because racial categories continue to have both political and psycho-logical importance that we continue (in keeping with many other researchers) to use the term 'race'. However, in keeping with newer theorisations, we also use 'racialised' and 'racialisation' to signal that the terms associated with 'race' represent social constructions rather than biological realities.

Terminology in the area of 'race' is constantly changing, and it is easy for both black and white people to use terms that some black people find offensive. In order to avoid anachronisms, when describing or quoting the work of earlier authors we use their terms. In describing our own research and views we refer to people with one white and one African or African Caribbean parent as of mixed parentage, and to those with two African or African Caribbean parents as black. In keep-ing with common usage, we do not, in the context of this book, call people of mixed parentage or of Asian origin black.

Some people may consider that too much is currently made of find-ing the right terms to refer to groups of people. However, the enormous amount of work now done on language and discourse makes it clear that what we call people affects the way in which we construct them. This is demonstrated by the example of social work interpretations of where it is appropriate to place children of mixed parentage. From the 1980s to the end of the twentieth century, social services departments tended to interpret their 'same-race placement' policy to mean that mixed-parentage children in care must be placed with black or mixed couples only. This was on the grounds that they cannot acquire a posi-tive black identity in a white family. This policy makes a number of assumptions that we set out to explore in the research reported in this book. In particular we wanted to find out how young people of mixed black and white parentage living with their own parents define their racial identity, what they feel about it, their attitudes and allegiance to black and white people and cultures, and their experience of, and ways of coping with, racism. We also wanted to analyse the factors that seemed to influence the young people's identities, and in particular the influence of the colour of the parents they lived with. We explored the same topics with a sample of their parents. Because a larger proportion of children of mixed African Caribbean and white origins enter care than any other racial group, we selected this group for study rather than, for example, those of mixed Asian and white origin.

Because this book is addressed to a wide public, we have placed statistical data in the Appendix. In this book we have quoted extensively from interview transcripts, so that the young people's voices can be heard.

2   People of mixed black and white parentage in Britain

A brief history

People with one white parent, and one black parent of African or African Caribbean descent, with whom this book is concerned, have long been part of British society. However, although there are a number of excellent histories of black people in Britain (e.g. Fryer, 1984; Ramdin, 1987; Shyllon, 1977; Walvin, 1973), no separate history of people of mixed black and white parentage has been written. In this sense, as a group they have no past, and no heroes or heroines with whom to identify. Yet although their fortunes have been intimately linked with those of other black people, their experiences have not always been the same. In a context in which it is increasingly being asserted that people of mixed parentage have a separate identity, it seems important to tease apart their history. In this chapter we briefly recount their history in Britain, and describe some eminent people of mixed parentage in the past, drawing on scattered passages in Fryer, Shyllon, Ramdin and others, and on original sources. We go on to discuss the changing attitudes of white people to those of mixed parentage over the centuries.

The age of slavery

In 1578, soon after the first Africans reached Britain, the first mixed marriages took place (Shyllon, 1977: 3). For the next 200 years, black slaves were brought to England in increasing numbers. Most were concentrated in London, but they were also numerous in the slave ports of Bristol and Liverpool, and could be found throughout Britain. It is impossible to calculate with any accuracy the size of the black population, but most historians have accepted the estimate of between 14,000 and 15,000 slaves made in the judgment in the Somerset case of 1772, when Lord Mansfield ruled that slaves could not lawfully be shipped out of England against their will. To this figure must be added an unknown number of freed slaves (Walvin, 1973: 46).

Since the great majority of the slaves brought here were males (a reflection of the demand for black footmen and male servants), sexual relationships and marriages with white women must have been frequent. Of the handful of freed slaves, such as Ottobah Cugoano and Olaudah Equiano, who became famous in the eighteenth century as writers and leaders of the black community, almost all married white women, but we know little about their children. We know even less about the great majority of mixed marriages, and their offspring, since both partners were poor, and usually servants. Some idea of the hardship of their lives may be obtained from an account of the life of a freed slave, Ukawsaw Gronniosaw, 'committed to paper by the elegant pen of a young lady of the town of Leominster' in 1770 (Fryer, 1984: 89).

Gronniosaw probably aroused her interest because he was the grandson of a king in what is now Nigeria, kidnapped by slave traders at the age of 15. Freed by his first master, who sent him to school, he worked as a servant, then served in the British Army, and on his discharge married a weaver called Betty, a poor English widow with a child. After working as a labourer on the roads in Colchester, he was unemployed during a severe winter, when the family survived only on charity, unable to afford a fire. Subsequently he obtained intermittent labouring work, and Betty hired a loom and wove. But when their three children became ill with smallpox they fell into arrears with their rent, and were saved from eviction only by a gift from a Quaker. Later, again falling into debt, they had to pawn their clothes and sell all their possessions. When the narrative ends, they were living on charity, and on Betty's earnings from weaving, since Gronniosaw was too ill to work. It is not known whether any of the children survived to adulthood – the death of one is recorded – or what became of them.

The only well-known person of mixed parentage in this period was George Bridgetower, born in 1779, son of an Austrian woman and a Barbadian, who was valet to an Austrian prince. The difference between his life and that of Gronniosaw is immense. George was a musical prodigy, who was brought by his father to play before the British King and Queen at the age of 9. Impressed by his talents and personality, the Prince of Wales took him under his protection, and appointed tutors to continue his education. He became famous throughout Europe as a concert violinist, and developed a friendship with Beethoven, who wrote the 'Kreutzer' sonata for him. This work was originally dedicated to him, but Beethoven subsequently changed the dedication after the two men quarrelled. His life and those of eminent black people of the period are recounted in Shyllon's *Black People in Britain* (1977).

People of mixed parentage during the nineteenth century

During the nineteenth century, following the abolition of the British slave trade in 1807, black immigration almost came to a halt, and the descendants of the freed slaves in Britain were absorbed into the general population. Occasionally, one of their descendants achieved some eminence. Thomas Birch Freeman, for example, a distinguished Methodist missionary, was the son of a 'full Negro', descended from a slave, who worked as a gardener on a country estate. His mother was a white servant in the same household. He himself married a white woman before setting sail for Nigeria in 1842, where he pioneered West African mission work (Ajayi, 1965).

However, most of the eminent people of mixed parentage during the nineteenth century were the West Indian-born 'mulatto' offspring of well-to-do white men. Compared to British-born people of mixed parentage at this time, they received a relatively good start in life. Early in the century two such men, William Davidson and Robert Wedderburn, threw in their lot with the fragmentary British revolutionary working-class movement. This movement sprang up after the Napoleonic War in response to widespread poverty and brutal government repression. Most of its leaders eventually suffered imprisonment, transportation or execution. Davidson, born in 1786, the son of the white Attorney-General of Jamaica and a black Jamaican, was sent to Britain to study law. After running away to sea, he returned to England to train and work as a cabinet maker. He married an English woman and taught at a Wesleyan Sunday school. Already a radical, his serious involvement in politics seems to have begun in 1819, in response to the Peterloo massacre, in which eleven unarmed demonstrators were killed and 500 injured in charges by armed militia. All over England groups of militant radicals began to prepare for action; it was widely believed that the country was on the verge of insurrection. Davidson and his friends decided to kill the members of the Cabinet as they dined together, an act they expected to lead to a general uprising. The plan was betrayed by a government spy and *agent provocateur*, and Davidson and four of his fellow conspirators were hanged (Stanhope, 1962).

The crowd was the largest that had ever turned out for an execution, and contingents of life-guards and artillery men were present in case of a rescue attempt. At his trial, it is noteworthy that Davidson based his defence on his traditional rights as an Englishman. It was, he argued, an ancient custom for the English:

> with arms to stand and claim their rights as Englishmen . . . And our history goes on further to say, that when another of their Majesties, the Kings of England, tried to infringe upon those rights, the people armed, and told him that if he did not give them the privileges of Englishmen, they would compel him by the point of the sword.

Davidson died bravely. He 'ascended the scaffold with a firm step, calm deportment, and undismayed countenance. . . . His conduct altogether was equally free from the appearance of terror, and the affectation of indifference' (Fryer, 1984: 219).

Robert Wedderburn, another leader in the struggle against the despotic government of the time, was born in Jamaica in 1762, the son of a wealthy Scottish sugar planter and a black slave. He came to Britain when he was 17, serving on a warship before becoming a tailor, and subsequently a Unitarian preacher. In 1817 he became involved with a group of socialist revolutionaries, known as Spenceans. He wrote numerous religious and revolutionary pamphlets, copies of which he sent to Jamaica, hoping for a simultaneous revolt of the white poor in Britain and the black slaves of the West Indies. Like Davidson, after the Peterloo massacre he believed that revolution was imminent, and urged the audiences he addressed, 'Arm and be ready, the day is near at hand'. Unlike Davidson, however, he did not become involved in actually planning an insurrection, and thus escaped execution, although he was imprisoned (Ramdin, 1987: 20).

Much better known was Mary Seacole, who was born in Jamaica in 1805, the daughter of a Scottish army officer and a Jamaican boarding-house keeper and 'doctress'. From her mother she learned both traditional herbal remedies and elements of Western medicine. Her expertise was considerably greater than that of Western nurses. As well as devising her own medicines, she had no hesitation in performing an autopsy, and stitching wounds and split ears. Mary, a woman of extraordinary courage and enterprise, had, like other remarkable women of the time, a passion for adventurous travel on her own. On her travels she nursed the sick in cholera and yellow fever epidemics, supporting herself by opening boarding-houses and restaurants for working men.

When the Crimean War broke out in 1854, Mary, then aged 49, volunteered her services to the British Army. When this offer was turned down because of racial prejudice, she decided to go to the

Crimea at her own expense, and to fund her nursing activities by selling meals and supplies to the troops. Besides tending the sick and wounded who came to her store, she would make her way under fire to the front line, with one mule carrying food and drink, and a second, bandages and medicines (Seacole, 1984). Fryer (1984:249) quotes from the memoirs of a lieutenant in the 63rd (West Suffolk) regiment:

> All the men swore by her, and in case of any malady would seek her advice and use her herbal medicines, in preference to reporting themselves to their own doctors. That she did effect some cures is beyond doubt, and her never failing presence among the wounded after a battle and assisting them made her beloved by the rank and file of the whole army.

After the war Mary Seacole was awarded four medals. *The Times*, having discovered that the Crimean venture had bankrupted her, appealed for funds on her behalf, as did *Punch*, and a four-day music festival was organised to raise money for her. She settled in England, published a bestselling autobiography, worked as a masseuse, and died in London in 1881. During the first part of the nineteenth century there were other West Indians of mixed parentage who settled in Britain, distinguished by wealth rather than achievement. These were the offspring of rich white West Indian planters and black women, sent to England to be educated and 'finished'. They were depicted in several contemporary novels. Jane Austen describes one such heiress, Miss Lambe, in *Sanditon*, an unfinished novel, written in 1817. Miss Lambe had brought her own maid with her to boarding-school, was given the best room, and 'was always of first consequence in any plan' of the proprietor. Another heiress was depicted by Thackeray in *Vanity Fair* (1848) – Miss Swartz, the daughter of a German slave trader and a slave. On leaving her English boarding-school she was presented at court, entertained by the aristocracy, and sought after by a prosperous merchant as a desirable match for his son.

Other black immigrants during the eighteenth and nineteenth centuries included small numbers of West Africans who came to Britain for their higher education, funded by wealthy parents or missionary societies. While few settled in Britain, some married white women and fathered children here. One such child was Samuel Coleridge-Taylor (named after the poet), who was born in 1875, and grew up to become a famous composer and conductor. His father, a Sierra Leonean, studied medicine in London, and married an English woman, who was working as a lady's companion. After qualifying, he tried to set up in general practice in Croydon, but was unable to attract patients. He returned to Sierra Leone without his wife and child, and died a few years later, leaving Samuel to be brought up by his mother and an English stepfather, described by Samuel's biographer as a 'working man'.

Samuel's musical talent was noticed and fostered by his teachers from an early age, and his choirmaster paid his fees to the Royal College of Music. By the age of 23 he was already famous for his choral-orchestral composition, *Hiawatha's Wedding Feast*; another cantata, *A Tale of Old Japan*, became equally popular. From his student days, it was his ambition to 'do for negro music what Brahms has done for Hungarian folk-music'; themes from negro hymns and songs figured frequently in his compositions, including the symphonic poem *Toussaint l'Ouverture*, and *Symphonic Variations on an African Air*. He died at the age of 37, at the height of his powers (Sayers, 1915).

By the end of the nineteenth century there were very few black people living in Britain, apart from West African and West Indian seamen who had settled in the dockland areas of the major ports. The descendants of the black slaves in Britain had 'disappeared' in the course of the century through intermarriage with white people. Certainly, the mixed-parentage men whom we know about in this period, such as Coleridge-Taylor and Thomas Birch Freeman, themselves married white women. (Mary Seacole seems not to have had children.) Many English people today must, unknowingly, have an African ancestor.

For more historical biographies of famous people of mixed parentage (including some discussed above) see Hoyles and Hoyles (1999). The biographies they present include Bob Marley, Mary Seacole, Samuel Coleridge-Taylor, the composer, and Frederick Douglas, as well as Arthur Wharton, the first black professional footballer and Ellen Craft, a runaway and slave.

Mixed black and white relationships and mixed parentage in the twentieth century

A second phase of black settlement in Britain began towards the end of the nineteenth century when West Indian and African seamen began to settle in the dockland area of several ports, the largest settlements being in Cardiff and Liverpool. Almost all the marriages they made must have been with white women. The 1911 Census found 9189 people born in the West Indies (some of whom would have been white) living in Britain. The two world wars brought a massive increase in their numbers, and presumably in the number of black-white relationships. But these increases were short-lived. As soon as the wars were over, and the

West Indians no longer required in the forces and industry, a hostile environment led most to accept repatriation to the West Indies (Walvin, 1973).

However, only a few years after the Second World War, the British postwar shortage of labour, coupled with large-scale unemployment in the West Indies, led many to return to Britain. At first this immigration was only a trickle, of several hundred a year: in 1951, according to the Census, only 15,000 West Indians were living in Britain, mainly in Cardiff and Liverpool (Walvin, 1973). This is the same number as the estimate for the black slave population of Britain in 1772. Indeed, since the total population in 1772 was about nine million, at that time they constituted a much larger proportion of society.

The situation changed dramatically when the third, and largest, phase of black settlement began in the mid-1950s, to be virtually ended by the Commonwealth Immigration Act of 1962. In 1954, the year of the first large-scale immigration, 24,000 West Indians arrived in Britain; in 1961, the final year in which immigration was unrestricted, the number was 61,600 (Rose and associates, 1969). The best government estimate of the current size of the 'West Indian' population (which includes those born here) is 428,000 (Haskey, 1991). Although this number is very large in comparison with any previous period, it still constitutes only 0.9 per cent of the British population, and 19 per cent of the ethnic minority population in Britain. The general belief that people of West Indian origin are far more numerous than this probably derives from the fact that they tend to live in a few centres, predominantly in London, with Birmingham as the second largest centre.

There are no British statistics on the frequency of intermarriage and mixed-parentage children before 1979. Evidence from the USA (Spickard, 1989) suggests that several factors influence the frequency of 'outmarriage' by members of a minority group. If the group is small or dispersed or the sex ratio unbalanced, 'outmarriage' is likely to be high – an isolated male is much more likely to marry into the majority group than one living in a large minority-group community. But these factors may be counterbalanced by others. The frequency of outmarriage tends to increase in successive generations, with very few of the first generation intermarrying. This increase is probably linked to a greater acceptance of the minority group by the majority, and to improvements in the economic status of the minority group (Spickard, 1989: 7).

In Britain, from the beginning of the twentieth century until the 1950s, the few West Indian immigrants were almost entirely male, and intermarriages were frequent. During the 1950s and 1960s the number of West Indian immigrants greatly increased, and included many single women, as well as the wives and children of men who had arrived a little earlier. By 1965 the numbers of West Indian men and women in Britain equalised for the first time, and a decline in the proportion of mixed marriages may have occurred. However, it increased later in the century, as indicated by Labour Force Surveys (annual sample surveys, which ask about the economic activity (or inactivity) and the ethnic origin of all members of the household) from the 1970s onwards. For percentages of black and Asian populations to be large enough to be calculated statistically, the findings from different years of the Labour Force Survey are combined. Analyses of the combined results for the Labour Force Surveys of 1979 and 1981 found that of 'West Indian' people (including those born in this country) who were married or cohabiting, 22 per cent of men and 10 per cent of women had a white partner. The corresponding figures for the 1989 survey were 24 per cent of men and 18 per cent of women (Owen, personal communication).

It seems likely that this increase is related to the changes in interracial attitudes which we document at the end of this chapter. It contrasts strongly with the position in the USA, where in 1980 only 3.6 per cent of black (African American) men and 1.2 per cent of black women were married to white people (Spickard, 1989). (On the other hand, nearly half of Japanese Americans and Native Americans had made outmarriages.) In Britain, men of West Indian origin were slightly less likely than men of African origin to marry white women, but they were three times more likely to do so than men from South Asia (Indians, Pakistanis, and Bangladeshis) (Coleman, 1985).

A further analysis of the data from the 1987 to 1989 surveys, carried out by Charlie Owen for this study, shows that a marked change in the sex ratio of black–white marriages is taking place in the younger generation, with equal proportions of young 'West Indian' men and women having white partners. Of 'West Indians' *under the age of 30* who were married or cohabiting, 27 per cent of men and 28 per cent of women had a white partner. This is an interesting development, and again suggests that a change in interracial attitudes is affecting marriage patterns. In many minority groups, even when the sex ratio is approximately equal, it is predominantly men rather than women who make outmarriages. This is the case with the Irish in Britain, and with black and Jewish people in the USA. In other US minority groups, notably Japanese, Chinese and Mexican Americans, it has been predominantly the women who married white people (Spickard, 1989). Spickard argues that these differences are related to differences in the images which men and women in the minority and majority groups have of each other. Since there has been virtually no research on this topic in

Britain, it is impossible to know whether this theory can explain the change in marriage patterns that we have noted above.

One consequence of the recent increase in interracial marriages is that the proportion of young children of mixed black and white parentage in the community is substantially larger than the proportion of teenagers. Indeed, of all the mixed white and African Caribbean *people* in this country, including both adults and children, *more than half* are under the age of 10. (The corresponding proportion for people with two black parents is 15 per cent; for those with two white parents, 12 per cent) (Coleman, 1985).

There is no information available about the social class of those who intermarry. In the past they are believed to have been predominantly drawn from the working class, but there is no evidence as to whether this was in fact the case, and whether it is so today. In the United States, the 1970 census found that the majority of intermarriages between black African Americans and white people were between well-educated members of the middle class. The same trend was present among Jewish and Japanese Americans (Spickard, 1989).

Current trends in mixed relationships and mixed parentage

Prior to the 1991 Census, the main source of data on Britain's minority ethnic populations had been the Labour Force Survey (Owen, 1993). The 1991 Census became the main source because it aims to enumerate the entire population and so should provide more complete data than do surveys, although it was very limited in the information it provided on mixed ethnic backgrounds. In fact, there is only one published table from the 1991 Census that includes any data on mixed parentage. From secondary analyses of these data, Charlie Owen found that:

> There were 54,569 people identified as *Black-White* (including those of African, African Caribbean and Other Black origin): this amounted to less than one tenth of 1 per cent of the population, or 994 persons per million. . . . There were 61,874 people identified as *Asian-White*: this is just over one tenth of 1 per cent, or, more precisely, 1,127 persons per million. . . . Finally there is a group of 112,061 labelled as *Other Mixed*, approximately 0.2 per cent of the population or 2,042 persons per million. Out of a total population for Great Britain of nearly 55 million, these three mixed groups – *Black-White*, *Asian-White* and *Other Mixed* – combined amount to less than half of one per cent.

> (Phoenix and Owen, 1996).

Although this may seem a very small percentage, it amounts to 8 per cent of all those who were classified in categories other than 'white'. Those who are included in the mixed category tend to have a younger age profile than those in other groups. This indicates that in 1991 mixed parentage was becoming increasingly common.

While an increase in those of mixed parentage does not necessarily entail an increase in mixed cohabiting or marital relationships, analyses done on the Labour Force Survey indicate that such relationships are increasing (Owen, 1993). There are no published tables in the Census on the ethnic groups of couples but, using the Census Sample of Ano-nymised Records (which records basic demographic data from a sample of those enumerated in 1991), it becomes clear that mixed relationships are proportionally more common among black and Asian people than among white people. This is hardly surprising, given that white people constitute 95 per cent of the British population: Over 99 per cent of *White* men and women living with a partner had a *White* partner. There are, however, gender differences in mixed relationships for black and Asian people. As described above, black men were more likely to have a white partner than were black women. The percentages of rela-tionships with *White* partners for the three South Asian groups were much lower. Of *Indian* men in couples, about 8 per cent had a *White* partner, 6 per cent of Pakistani men and 3 per cent of Bangladeshi men. The order was the same for women but the percentages were all lower. For the *Chinese* and *Other Groups–Other Asian* the percentages were higher, and higher for women than for men: a quarter of *Chinese* women in couples were with a *White* partner. (Phoenix and Owen, 1996: 120)

In the USA, there has also been an increase in the numbers of those who identify themselves as 'biracial' and in 'interracial marriages' (Root, 1996, 2001). Qian (1997: 263) analysed data from the 1980 and 1990 US Censuses. He found that

> rarely, but increasingly between 1980 and 1990, interracial marriage of whites occurs most frequently with Asian Americans (who are Japanese, Chinese, Korean etc. rather than Indian, Pakistani or Bangladeshi as in Britain), followed by Hispanics, and then by African Americans.

The 2000 US Census found that seven million people (2.4 per cent of the population) identified themselves as belonging simultaneously to two racialised groupings. 'The Census Bureau predicts that there will be many more mixed-race people in the future' (*The Economist*, 2001: 55). This is particularly the case since nearly half of those who chose the 'mixed' category were under 18 years of age – although it may be that older and younger people of mixed parentage were answering the questions in different ways.

At the time of writing, analyses from the UK Census in 2001 are not yet available. However, on the basis of his analyses of data from the Policy Studies Institute Fourth National Survey of Ethnic Minorities and of the Labour Force Survey, Richard Berthoud (1999) has suggested that it may be the case that the majority of Caribbean men who are embarking on cohabitation or marriage in the twenty-first century have white women partners. From the combined Labour Force Survey of 1992 to 1995, Berthoud argues that increases in mixed parentage amongst *British born* people of Caribbean origin will mean an increase in the number of people who have some Caribbean background, and a reduction in the number who have two parents of Caribbean background. His analyses indicate that half of the *British-born* men of Caribbean origin and one third of the *British-born* women who are married or cohabiting are living with a white partner. The rate of mixed partnership is increasing more rapidly for men of African Caribbean origin than for women (Berthoud, 2001). The findings from the Fourth National Survey indicate that marriage and cohabitation with white people were much less common among South Asians than among Caribbeans (Modood *et al.*, 1994, 1997). About one in five *British-born* men of Indian or African Asian origin surveyed had a white wife; one in ten Indian or African Asian women had white live-in partners, while very few Bangladeshi- and Pakistani-origin people had mixed relationships with white people.

In summary, then, those data available indicate that there are a growing number of people in racially mixed relationships and marked increases in the number of people of mixed parentage. Thus, despite negative constructions of mixed parentage, many people are contesting the social proscription on crossing constructed racialised boundaries. The demographic data provide the context within which it is possible to understand ideological and discursive shifts with regard to mixed parentage.

While demographic data are interesting in themselves, it is important to note that the classifications used as the basis of demographic analyses are themselves socially constructed. Decisions about which analyses to perform are not (in keeping with the production of other knowledge) objective and decontextualised (Owen, 2001) but informed by sociopolitical interests. The fact that the demography of race is a contentious issue is well demonstrated by the furore generated by (the now successful) calls for a mixed category in the 2000 US Census (see Root, 1996). It is therefore important that, with the inclusion of a mixed question in both the US Census in 2000 and the UK Census in 2001, there is continued debate about which analyses are most helpful.

White people's attitudes to people of mixed black and white parentage

Up to the mid-nineteenth century: a complex of attitudes

Attitudes to people of mixed black and white parentage were very different in Britain, the USA, and the West Indies. In the West Indies a three-caste system operated. Because there were very few white women available, settled concubinage between white planters and black slaves was an open and common practice. Their offspring constituted a separate caste, with a status intermediate between black and white. They were usually free, often well educated, and worked as overseers, teachers, clerks, skilled tradesmen, or even slave-holding planters. From the 1730s the Jamaican legislature passed numerous private acts conferring on the 'mulatto' offspring of individual planters the rights and privileges of white people, including the right to inherit. Thackeray's depiction of one such heiress in *Vanity Fair* has already been mentioned. However, as a group they had few civil rights, and were despised by many white people, although often envied by black people.

In the USA their situation was much less favourable. There was no shortage of white women, and open cohabitation between white masters and black slaves was rare. Instead, there was clandestine concubinage and forced sex between white masters and women slaves. In the southern states the majority of their offspring lived out their lives as slaves, often with no special privileges. However, in certain cities, for example, New Orleans and Charleston, and on some of the 'great plantations', freed mulattos, often well educated and even wealthy, formed a separate caste, as in the West Indies. They typically married other mulattos, and in order to maintain their privileged status shunned the company of darker-skinned people. As in the West Indies, gradations according to the proportion of 'white blood' were recognised, from 'mulatto' (one black parent) through 'quadroon' (one black grandparent) to 'octoroon' (one black great grandparent). In the north, too, free mulattos assumed a superior status to black people. In Philadelphia they formed their own church, to which black people were not admitted.

After the emancipation of the slaves, the USA shifted to a two-caste system. The 'one drop' rule prevailed; that is, anyone with any known negro ancestry, even if it was one great-grandparent, was classified as black. However, until the 1960s lighter skins and 'Caucasian' features continued to give prestige in the black community, and sometimes led to preferential treatment by white people. According to Spickard (1989), whereas white people saw only negroes, black people saw dozens of gradations, from 'ash black' to 'olive brown' to 'high yeller'. Nevertheless, while lighter skins gave status, 'high yellows' often carried the stigma of illegitimacy. Since the census count of mulattos increased steadily after 1850, it is likely that interracial sexual mixing continued, together with a progressive lightening of black Americans, through intermarriage between people of lighter skins. Interracial marriages, however, were rare. Thirty out of forty-eight states retained laws against racial intermarriage until after the Second World War, and it was only in 1967 that the US Supreme Court finally put an end to such laws.

People of mixed parentage fascinated American novelists. Definite stereotypes of them emerged, quite different from the stereotypes of the 'negro'. Before the abolition of slavery, men of mixed parentage were often portrayed by Abolitionist novelists, such as Harriet Beecher Stowe, as tragic heroes. Typically, they were depicted as the all-but-white, handsome, intelligent offspring of southern white gentlemen and black or 'mulatto' slaves. Rebelling against their fate as slaves, they either escaped to freedom or were killed in the attempt (Berzon, 1978).

In Britain, the only people of mixed parentage with whom novelists were concerned, and then rarely, were West Indian heiresses, whose role, far from being tragic, was to throw a comic sidelight on the cupidity of society. In Jane Austen's unfinished novel *Sanditon* (1817), Lady Denham was anxious that her impoverished nephew, Sir Edward, should court Miss Lambe, a 'mulatto' heiress, about whom nothing was known except that she was rich. In Thackeray's *Vanity Fair* (1848), Mr Osborne and his daughters were desperate for a 'mulatto' heiress, Miss Swartz, to marry into the family. Insofar as these heiresses were given 'racial' characteristics, they were the contemporary stereotypical characteristics attributed to black people, rather than any specific to those of mixed parentage. Thackeray, for example, depicts Miss Swartz as simple to the point of being ridiculous, and lacking in taste and refinement, although affectionate and good natured. British-born people of mixed parentage did not arouse the interest of novelists, perhaps because they were very few in number, and both their parents were usually poor, and often servants.

So far as can be judged, for much of this period attitudes to people of mixed parentage in Britain did not differ from the prevailing attitudes to people with two black parents. These attitudes were more varied and complex than those in the USA, and changed over time. Initially, perceptions of them were influenced by the ancient, pre-Christian association between blackness and sin, and by the fact that they were regarded as heathens (Barker, 1978). By the mid-eighteenth century British ships were transporting tens of thousands of Africans to the West Indies each year. They became familiar as slaves, and the stereotype of the slave – as someone of limited intelligence, irresponsible and lazy, who stole, lied, and was treacherous and superstitious – joined or replaced earlier images of heathen savages. The most notorious and eloquent apologist for the planters, Edward Long, in his *Candid Reflections* (1772), advanced 'scientific' reasons for justifying slavery, on the grounds that black and white people belong to different species, that hybrids between them are eventually infertile, and that black people are closer to apes than man.

Like all 'biological' racists, Long was bitterly opposed to mixed black and white unions, and infuriated by the number he observed in England.

> The lower class of women in England are remarkably fond of the blacks, for reasons too brutal to mention; they would connect themselves with horses and asses, if the laws permitted them. By these ladies they generally have a numerous brood. Thus in the course of a few generations more the English blood will be so contaminated with this mixture . . . till the whole nation resembles the Portuguese and the Moriscos in complexion of skin and baseness of mind.
>
> (Walvin, 1973: 52)

William Cobbett, too, observed in 1804 that a 'shocking number of English women were prepared to accept not only black lovers, but much worse, black husbands' (Walvin, 1973: 181). Olaudah Equiano, a black leader who himself married an English woman, wrote to the *Public Advertiser* in reply to one such outburst, pointing out that in the West Indies white men fathered 'mulatto' children with impunity. But, he went on:

> Why not establish intermarriages at home, and in our Colonies?

and encourage open, free and generous love, upon Nature's own wide and extensive plan, subservient only to moral rectitude, without distinction of the colour of a skin?

(Shyllon, 1977: 41)

There is no doubt that Long's belief that black people were sub-human was shared by many British people. It was entirely consistent with the fact that black people had been treated like animals for 200 years, especially in the West Indies. However, not all, and perhaps not the majority of British people shared these attitudes. John Wesley, for example, argued that the supposedly inborn characteristics of the slave were produced by slavery.

> Are not stubbornness, cunning, pilfering, and diverse other vices the natural fruits of slavery? You keep them stupid and wicked, by cutting them off from all opportunities of improving, either in knowledge or virtue. And now you assign their want of wisdom and goodness as the reason for using them worse than brutes.
>
> (Walvin, 1973: 181)

Abolitionists did not all believe in the equality of black and white people. To some, they were innocent children of nature, corrupted by Europeans. Others, while accepting that black people were inferior, argued that this could be changed by education.

It is impossible to assess the extent of the support for these different points of view. We know that some British people educated and freed their slaves, and left them money in their wills; others subscribed to the rescue of slaves from their owners, and to the legal costs of defending slaves in court. The London 'mob' was notorious for concealing runaway slaves, and black people became leaders of sectors of the radical working-class movement. Some English people, such as Granville Sharp, worked tirelessly to help individual slaves, and for the abolition of slavery. Many English women had black husbands and lovers. Lord Mansfield, the Lord Chief Justice in the Somerset case of 1772, referred to above, brought up the West Indian-born mixed-parentage daughter of his nephew with his own children in London, and left her a legacy in his will (Shyllon, 1977). Individual black people of eminence were respected and befriended in intellectual circles, and wealthy black people moved in the highest social circles. Shyllon quotes a contemporary author who contrasts attitudes to people of mixed parentage in England and the West Indies (Shyllon, 1977: 59):

If a white and a brown child should be sent to Europe at the same time, and educated together at the same school, though they be in habits of the greatest intimacy while there, they discontinue that intimacy on their return to the West Indies . . . the white Miss no longer recognises her quondam companion and schoolfriend as an equal. . . . It is a pity that a parent, after having bestowed on his offspring a genteel and liberal education, in a country where at least they experience a respect and attention equal to their merits, should suffer them to be brought back to one where their feelings . . . are perpetually liable to be wounded by contumely.

While the friendly relationships that sometimes took place in England between black and white people would have been impossible in racially stratified societies such as the West Indies or the USA, there was certainly a good deal of racism around, quite apart from the presence of slavery. Sancho, for example, a respected black eighteenth-century writer, clearly took this for granted. In his *Letters* he describes a visit to the Vauxhall pleasure gardens as follows: 'We went by water – had a coach home – were gazed at – followed etc. etc. – but not much abused.' William Clarkson, an English Abolitionist who entertained the former Queen of Haiti and her two daughters in his home for several months in 1821, noted that 'there was a sort of shrink at admitting them into high society' (Shyllon, 1977: 72). William Davidson, the mixed-parentage revolutionary leader, expressed anxiety at his trial that he would not be given a fair trial because of his colour.

Mary Seacole, the 'mulatto' West Indian nurse, while beloved by her patients, and eventually regarded as a national heroine, initially found herself blocked by racial discrimination. Attempting to follow Florence Nightingale to the Crimea, she was told by the lady in charge of recruiting that no more nurses were required.

'I read in her face, [she wrote] that had there been a vacancy I should not have been chosen to fill it. . . . Doubts and suspicions arose in my heart for the first and last time, thank Heaven. Was it possible that American prejudices against colour had some root here? Did these ladies shrink from accepting my aid because my blood flowed beneath a somewhat duskier skin than theirs? Tears streamed down my foolish cheeks, as I stood in the fast-thinning streets'.

However, the indomitable Mary was not long downcast. 'A good night's rest served to strengthen my determination. Let what might happen, to the Crimea I would go.' (Seacole, 1984: 125)

As the nineteenth century advanced, the black population in Britain declined, but racist views became more widespread. In 1833 the black American Shakespearean actor, Ira Aldridge, who settled in England, was the butt of scurrilous attacks by critics. The *Athenaeum* thought it 'impossible that Mr Aldridge should fully comprehend the meaning and force of even the words he utters' and protested 'in the name of propriety and decency against a lady-like girl like Miss Ellen Tree being pawed about on the stage by a black man' (Fryer, 1984: 254). Nevertheless, such attitudes were still not universal, and Aldridge played to packed houses in the provinces for another twenty years before abandoning Britain for the continent, where he met with universal acclaim. A similar mixture of attitudes is depicted by Thackeray in *Vanity Fair* (1848) where, as described above, the father and sisters were anxious to welcome a West Indian heiress into the family for the sake of her money, but the son refused to comply. 'Marry that mulatto woman? I don't like the colour, sir. Ask the black that sweeps opposite Fleet Street, sir. I'm not going to marry a Hottentot Venus.'

From the mid-nineteenth century to the First World War: 'scientific racism' triumphant

Until the mid-nineteenth century, the theory that black people were inherently inferior was by no means universally accepted. Many contemporary scientists and intellectuals attributed black 'inferiority' to environmental causes such as lack of education and Christian beliefs, ill-treatment, a hot climate and poor diet. Even dark skin pigmentation was thought to be a comparatively short-term result of climatic factors, which would disappear within a few generations of living in Europe (Barker, 1978). Nor did all pro-slavery writers use racist arguments. Some defended slavery solely in terms of economic expediency, or the rights of property owners, distancing themselves from the argument that black people were scarcely human. Hence 'gentlemanly', wealthy and eminent black people were generally treated with respect in the eighteenth and early nineteenth centuries, even though this might be mixed with uneasiness.

However, the climate of opinion changed from about the mid-nineteenth century. Heredity began to be seen as a far more important influence than environment on the human character. It became generally agreed, as it had not been formerly, that there were a variety of races with different inborn physical, intellectual and moral characteristics. The different skull shape of negroes was said to indicate their lower level of intelligence, hence attempts to educate them were regarded as futile. Long's theory that negroes are a distinct species, closer to the ape than the European, was revived. Although Darwin argued that there is only one human species, and that all human beings are descended from apelike ancestors, he nonetheless believed that natural selection had produced a range of races, varying from the primitive (a category in which he included the Irish as well as negroes) to the most evolved, the Anglo-Saxons.

Late nineteenth-century 'scientific racism' thus involved not only a belief in the superiority of white people, but of the Anglo-Saxon 'race' in particular. The theory provided a justification both for the expansion of colonialism that took place at this time, and for virulent discrimination against the Jewish and Irish 'races'. Racism permeated the press, fiction, popular culture and children's stories. 'Nigger minstrel' troupes (usually white performers, painted with a garish black countenance) perpetuated the stereotype of the happy-go-lucky, lazy, singing and dancing simpleton. Hardly any eminent British people came out openly against racism.

Those few black people who lived in Britain experienced a great deal of abuse. Samuel Coleridge-Taylor's father, though qualifying as a doctor in England, had to return to West Africa because he could not attract patients in England, and Samuel himself, who had a white mother, had to contend not only with everyday abuse in the streets, but also discrimination from part of the music establishment. According to his biographer, while some music critics of the time hailed him as a genius, many more suggested that such praise should be moderated, since people of negro blood never fulfil their early promise; his later works were 'consciously or unconsciously ignored by many who profess to shape musical opinion in this country' (Sayers, 1915: 106).

Thomas Birch Freeman, the Methodist missionary of mixed parentage referred to earlier, experienced the change of attitudes that took place during the century. His arrival in Nigeria in 1842 marked the effective beginning of missionary enterprise in that country. He set up and maintained a chain of missions and mission schools, and was described 'as an extraordinary man, a pious visionary, yet immensely practical'. Before his death in 1890, however, a reorganisation in the Nigerian missions took place. A new generation of white missionaries believed that Africans, without the benefit of centuries of Christian culture, could never achieve a civilised status; the 'African character' was said to be synonymous with lying, hypocrisy, drunkenness and immorality. African bishops were ousted, and African pastors were dismissed, or deprived of any power in the Church, and allocated a lower salary than the European pastors; there was debate about whether Freeman should be classified as a 'native' for this purpose. The earlier policy of encouraging the growth of an African middle class through education and promotion was overturned (Ajayi, 1965).

Hostility to mixed unions, an inherent part of 'scientific racism', became almost universal. Many scientists asserted that race mixture would lead to physical, mental and emotional deformities, or to 'hybrid degeneration'; that is, the offspring of the mixture would inherit none of the good qualities of either parent and would die off after a few generations. Sir Francis Galton, founder of the eugenics movement, argued that the English, as an intellectually superior race, should not breed with an inferior race such as negroes because the reduction in average intelligence that would result would cause an even greater reduction in the proportion of individuals in the highest grade of intelligence (Provine, 1973: 790).

Scientists' fears about the results of interracial unions were reflected in new stereotypes of 'mulattos' which appeared in American fiction. A popular theme involved the idea of racial atavism; that is, that despite the veneer of white civilisation, 'mixed bloods' were liable at any time to revert to the savage, primitive behaviour of the jungle. Another stereotype was 'the mixed blood' as a straightforward villain, the incarnation of evil, who combines the worst traits of both races. However, there were still frequent depictions of 'mulattos' as tragic figures, usually women, beautiful, intelligent and all-but-white, torn between the two strands of their ancestry. This conflict was usually seen in terms of a divided racial inheritance, a 'clash of blood' (Berzon, 1978).

Perhaps because almost all the few people of mixed parentage in Britain at this time belonged to the most deprived sector of society they seem to have played no part in British fiction, although Anglo-Indians were sometimes depicted. There was certainly no equivalent of the tragically beautiful heroine of American novels.

Attitudes since the First World War: 'eugenic racism' begins to give way to greater liberalism

The rise of the eugenics movement in the early years of the century seems to have led to people of mixed parentage being seen for the first time in Britain as having characteristics distinct from, and even more undesirable than, those of black people. According to a pre-Second World War writer (Dover, 1937: 279), it was believed that they were 'the work of the devil, that they inherit the vices of both parents and the virtues of neither, that they are without exception infertile, unbalanced, indolent, immoral, and degenerate'. The eugenics movement, from which these views originated, developed out of the new science of genetics. It was dedicated to applying the principles learned from animal and plant crossing to improving the 'human stock'. This was to be done by encouraging 'superior' people to breed, and by trying to prevent criminals, the mentally sick or unsound, and other undesirables, from reproducing. Racial intermarriage was to be discouraged, because of a belief that the new combinations of genetic traits that resulted would be disharmonious, or would weaken the white 'stock'. Davenport, a geneticist, and the leading advocate of eugenics in the United States, pointed to the example of unsuccessful animal cross-breeds as a warning of the dangers of racial mixing. When Leghorns, which laid eggs well, were crossed with Brahmas, which were good brooders, the hybrid offspring were failures both as egg layers and as brooders. Similarly, he argued, 'one often sees in mulattos an ambition and push combined with intellectual inadequacy which makes the unhappy hybrid dissatisfied with his lot and a nuisance to others' (Provine, 1973: 791).

As late as 1930 another leading geneticist, Herbert Jennings, argued that disharmonious physical combinations would result from human 'crosses' (Provine, 1973: 793). According to Provine, both Davenport and Jennings were staunch supporters of civil liberties, and opposed to race discrimination. They believed that their opposition to race mixing was based on objective scientific grounds. These grounds were undermined in the late 1920s when a number of studies of 'race crossing' in Hawaii, Pitcairn Island, Canada and the USA failed to discover physical disharmonies. But many geneticists continued to believe that race mixing resulted in *mental* disharmony, or neurosis, instancing the general belief at the time that 'mixed bloods' were irrational, moody and temperamental. Other geneticists continued to argue, as Galton had, that by 'crossing' with black people, whites would lose a sizeable proportion of their most intelligent people.

It was not until the mid-1930s that some leading biologists, shocked by Nazi race doctrines, argued that there was no evidence to substantiate these fears, and that 'if the alleged inferiority of half-castes really exists, it is much more likely to be the product of the unfavourable social atmosphere in which they grow up than to any effect . . . of their mixed heredity' (Huxley, 1936: 11). And it was not until the early 1950s that UNESCO issued a statement by geneticists and physical anthropologists that 'no biological justification exists for prohibiting intermarriages between persons of different races' and that 'available scientific knowledge provides no basis for believing that the groups of mankind differ in their innate capacity for intellectual and emotional development' (UNESCO, 1951: 15). Virtually all the leading biologists consulted agreed with the first statement, that race mixing is harmless, but by no means all were willing to subscribe to the statement about the intellectual equality of all races.

Studies carried out in Britain in the 1940s suggest that mixed-parentage people at that time suffered not only from the same double stigma as people with two black parents – that of colour and low social class – but also from the additional stigma of having a mother who was considered depraved. Little, for example, studied a 'coloured' community in Cardiff docklands in the early 1940s (Little, 1948) at a time when the two largest settled black communities in Britain were in Tiger Bay, Cardiff, and the South End of Liverpool. In these communities black seamen lived in houses of multiple occupancy with white women, who were said to be drawn from the lowest stratum of society. Virtually all the children in the community were of mixed parentage. On leaving school, because of the colour bar which then operated, and their poor educational qualifications, the girls found it almost impossible to obtain work; neither employers nor employees would accept them for factory work or domestic service. The boys, who might find employment at sea, or in dead-end jobs, for instance, as errand boys, fared only slightly better. The whole community was isolated by the colour bar, which prevented them from using clubs, dance-halls, restaurants, pubs, etc. in the rest of the city. Not surprisingly, the young people were said to 'act negatively', and to be unreliable and shiftless.

Collins (1957), who carried out field studies in black dockland communities between 1949 and 1951, found that 90 per cent of the West Indian men were married to white women, the rest to 'half-castes'. A mixed marriage was said to result in the estrangement of the woman from her family and friends. Reconciliation, partial or complete, might follow, but in the case of the few middle-class white families involved, this rarely happened.

Both Collins and Patterson (1963), who carried out field-work in Brixton in the 1950s, noted that, while marriages between white men and West Indian women were very unusual, when they did occur, they met with much less hostility than those between white women and West Indian men. Little (1948: 256) had also noted that 'prejudice is most quickly and emotionally aroused by relations between white females and coloured males'.

According to Patterson (1963: 283), a popular white view in Brixton in the late 1950s was that white girls were intrigued 'by the coloured man's reported sexual prowess and superior sexual equipment', a belief that has created anxiety among white men since at least the eighteenth century. An important cause of the 'race riots' in Cardiff and Liverpool in 1919, when black men were hunted down by gangs of white men, was said to have been white male anger at the liaisons between black men and white women which had developed during the First World War (Fryer, 1984: 302). The evidence certainly suggests that the objections to mixed unions arose as much from anxieties about black male sexuality as from worries about the offspring of the union. This was, of course, always the case in the United States, where a blind eye was turned to interracial sex and even marriage between white men and black women. Black men, on the other hand, were always seen as potential rapists, and lynchings for no more than asking a white woman for a date continued into the 1950s.

'Scientific' racism was, as we have described, discredited by many biologists in 1951, but the belief that black people belong to a different and inferior race, and that 'interbreeding' would harm the white race, lingered on in popular consciousness, and white–black marriages continued to be strongly disapproved of by many white people. Survey data are limited in that they often offer people predetermined attitudinal choices and cannot tell us much about why people gave the answers they did. However, since there are few in-depth studies on attitudes, survey data provide some insight into trends in thinking about mixed parentage. A Gallup poll in 1958 found that 71 per cent of respondents disapproved of mixed marriages, and only 13 per cent approved. A Gallup poll in the USA in the same year found that over 90 per cent disapproved (Spickard, 1989: 293). Patterson's field study in Brixton, carried out between 1955 and 1958, found that local attitudes to mixed relationships varied from the mildly disapproving to outright distaste: 'Disgusting. I don't know how a decent woman could let a blackie touch her' (1963: 282). She claims that few 'respectable' local white girls would be seen out with a West Indian.

The late 1960s saw the beginning of more liberal white attitudes. The proportion of people disapproving of marriages between 'whites and nonwhites' fell to 57 per cent in a 1968 Gallup poll, and to 42 per cent when the question was repeated in 1973. (The comparable proportions in the USA were 76 per cent and 65 per cent) (Spickard, 1989: 293). Nevertheless, in a study of mixed marriages in Brixton between 1970 and 1971 Benson found that white women who were sexually involved with black partners were still known as 'black men's women', and because of white hostility were forced to move into a black social world (Benson, 1981: 49).

More recent polls have shown a continued liberalisation of white attitudes. For example, on a number of occasions between 1983 and 1991 the British Social Attitudes Survey has asked respondents if they would mind if a close relative married someone of *Asian* origin or of *West Indian* origin. About half of the respondents said they would mind, either a lot or a little, although there has been a fall in the number who mind, from 54 per cent in 1983 to 43 per cent in 1991. The British Social Attitudes Survey of 1987 found that only 27 per cent of those polled would 'mind a lot' if one of their close relatives was to marry a person of West Indian origin, and a further 23 per cent would 'mind a little'. A survey carried out for the Runnymede Trust in 1991 included a less personally worded question: 'Do you agree or disagree that people should marry only within their own ethnic group?' Of the white respondents, 31 per cent agreed, or tended to agree, and 58 per cent disagreed (Amin *et al.*, 1991). Subsequent unpublished tables show that there was a marked tendency for younger respondents to have more liberal attitudes. Of those aged between 18 and 34, only 19 per cent agreed, or tended to agree, compared with 49 per cent of those aged 55 and over. Middle-class people had more liberal attitudes than working-class people.

In a poll conducted for the *Independent on Sunday* (7 July 1991), respondents were asked the extent to which they agreed or disagreed with the following statement: 'People should only marry people of their own ethnic group.' Among *white* respondents, 31 per cent said they agreed; 17 per cent of *black* respondents and 39 per cent of *Asian* respondents also agreed.

While there are many shortcomings of survey data, the fact that there is still opposition to black–white relationships was brought home to the British public by media accounts of attacks on black men with white girlfriends (see e.g. *Daily Mail*, 19 October 1993; *Guardian*, 10 June 1994; *Sun*, 21 June 1994; *Sun*, 23 September 1994). The fact that these publicised attacks were on black men with white girlfriends is probably not accidental since there is a long history of race and gender intersecting in opposition to mixed relationships. Opposition to mixed relationships is well known to people who are in such relationships since it has had a direct impact on many (EYTARN, 1995; Katz, 1996). From their conversations with people in mixed relationships, Alibhai-Brown and Montague (1992: 4) argue that:

'In a society where our reluctance to become "involved" leaves tor-tured children at risk in their own homes and raped women lying in gutters, perfect strangers think they have the right to abuse you, or your partner or your child, because you have different skin colours.'

Attitudes of black and Asian people to mixed marriages

Very little is known about the attitudes of black people to mixed marriages, and to the offspring of mixed marriages. Collins (1957), who carried out a field study in black docklands communities between 1949 and 1951, reported that women who had recently arrived from the West Indies objected to the mixed relationships which they found in Britain, on the grounds that the white women involved were of low class and dubious morals. In the 1970s, at the height of the black consciousness movement, many black people considered that sexual relationships with white people represented a denial of black identity, and the issue was much debated in the black press. However, as we have shown, the proportion of black people marrying or living with white people has steadily increased. The Runnymede Trust poll in 1991, reported above, found that the black respondents were less opposed to mixed relationships than the white: only 18 per cent agreed that people should marry only within their own ethnic group. The trend reported for the white respondents of the younger age groups and higher social classes to have more liberal attitudes was not present, but there was a marked tendency for fewer black men than women to oppose mixed relationships. These findings, together with the marked increase in the number of intermarriages, suggest that at the present time black attitudes to mixed marriages are in the main favourable.

The Fourth National Survey on ethnic minorities in Britain done by the Policy Studies Institute (Beishon *et al.*, 1998) provides further information. This found that people of South Asian origin (26 per cent) were less likely to say that most people from their ethnic group would be positive about mixed marriages than were white people (33 per cent), who in turn were less positive than people of Caribbean origin (57 per cent). Less than a quarter of South Asians said that most members of their group 'would not mind' if a close relative were to marry a white person. As we have seen, marriage and cohabitation with white people was much less common for South Asians than for Caribbeans (Modood *et al.*, 1994, 1997). However, when asked if they would personally mind if a close relative had a mixed marriage, 84 per cent of Caribbean, 72 per cent of white and almost half of the Asian sample said they would not mind. As in the Runnymede Trust poll, younger people were most likely to say they would not mind, with almost 90 per cent of Caribbean and white 16–34-year-olds saying they would not mind if a close rela-tive had a mixed marriage. On the whole, those without qualifications and in manual occupations said that they would mind more than would those with qualifications and in professional jobs. This was reversed for those of Caribbean origin (Modood, 1997).

However, some black people said that marrying into a white family is disloyal to one's origins and could be an opportunist move into white society (Beishon *et al.*, 1998; Modood *et al.*, 1994). From his analyses, Berthoud (2001) argues that suspicions that social mobility is a motive for black people marrying white partners are not borne out by the demographic data available. He found that mixed relationships were equally common among those with high and low levels of education, and among those with good and bad employment experiences. This picture may be rather different in the USA. From their analyses, Heaton and Albrecht (1996: 203) argue that 'people who intermarry, regardless of race or gender, tend to have higher educational and economic status than do those in homogamous marriages'. Neither set of analyses sup-ports ideas about mixed marriages being for reasons of social mobility.

What about the children?

While there has been a longstanding negative orientation to relation-ships between black and white people and the children from such unions, the nature of that negative orientation shifted in the last cen-tury. The change was from eugenic concerns with 'miscegenation' to liberal concerns about the welfare of the children born from such unions, i.e. to expressions of benevolent concerns about the children.

> Many people who are in almost all other respects very tolerant of coloured people defend their objection to mixed marriages on the grounds that the children of such marriages are bound to suffer.
>
> (Richmond, 1961: 284)

> The prevailing view of mixed race children is that they have identity problems because of their ambiguous social position . . . the stereotype of the 'tortured misfit'.
>
> (Wilson, 1987: 1–2)

Although this appears, at first sight, to be a benign shift, it is, in effect, also negative. This is because they still construct mixed relationships as problematic. The apparently benevolent concern with the welfare of children masks its deleterious effects in three related ways. Firstly, it prevents charges of racism by deflecting attention from racist discourses on to children of mixed parentage as misfits. Secondly, it individualises the issue by shifting focus on to the problems of identity for the children produced from mixed unions. Finally, it constructs 'regimes of truth' (Foucault, 1980) which are designed to lead to internal, individual regulation of mixed relationships since external controls are neither legal nor currently socially acceptable. Thus, since most parents do not have children with the intention of damaging them, the implication is that concerned, responsible parents should not produce children of mixed parentage. It can thus be used to warrant attempted deterrence of mixed relationships and intrusive comments to, or even physical violence on, those who become parents of mixed-parentage children (Alibhai-Brown, 2001; Alibhai-Brown and Montague, 1992).

Foreboding about the impact on children of being of mixed parentage may, of course, be well intentioned, as from the black psychiatrist Alvin Poussaint, who has specialised in the development of black children.

> Dr. Poussaint warns that Black-White individuals must realize that regardless of the chosen label, American society will continue treating them as Black people. 'Children should not be misled', he says. 'A new label will not keep other kids from taunting and calling them names.'
>
> (Norment, 1995: 112)

Yet such concern glosses over the fact that children of mixed parentage report that they are called racist names by black as well as white children. While they are certainly called names that black children are called, they are also called names specifically aimed at children who are of mixed parentage. In addition, those living with at least one white parent (about three-quarters of all the mixed groups (Owen, 2001)) often also have to recognise that other children find it difficult to accept that they have a white parent. While it could be argued that this simply makes children of mixed parentage more like black children – who would also not be expected to have white parents – it also differentiates them in that children with two black parents do not generally have to face this experience.

More worrying are reports that children of mixed parentage who live with lone white mothers are sometimes isolated in white racist contexts which psychologically damage them (Banks, 1992, 1996). It is, of course, appalling that children (or indeed adults) should have to face such circumstances and it is crucially important to address these politically, psychologically, and within childcare and social work. It is, however, important to contextualise these findings. Studies of 'mixed relationships' and 'mixed parentage' generally find that many of the white families into which children are born are hostile, or at least anxious, about their white relatives having children of mixed parentage (Alibhai-Brown, 2001; Alibhai-Brown and Montague, 1992; Early Years Trainers Anti-Racist Network (EYTARN) 1995). The children themselves are sometimes hurt by this awareness and, in some cases, grandparents continue to be hostile (EYTARN, 1995). In addition, some of the white parents who have children of mixed parentage are implicated in racist narratives in that they will, for example, sometimes hide their children or pretend that they are not theirs in response to racism – but in order to protect their feelings, rather than their children's safety (Ifekwunigwe, 1997; Mama, 1995). In addition, children of mixed parentage are more likely than white or black children to enter local authority care and be 'looked after' for longer periods (Bebbington and Miles, 1989). All these issues are likely to have far-reaching consequences for children.

In tackling these very real problems, however, it is important to bear in mind that, equally, many white parents of mixed parentage children make efforts to disrupt racism and racialised discourses, as do some of their parents and families (EYTARN, 1995; Katz, 1996). It would also be disingenuous to make the implicit assumption that black parents of black children are necessarily either positive about their children's blackness or antiracist (see e.g. Mama, 1995). Some black children growing up with black parents are also hurt by racism (as indicated by clinical reports of black children attempting to scrub their skins white or the use of bleach cream). Yet, as Mama (1995) points out, this hurt does not necessarily lead to permanent psychological damage. Racialised identities are continuously in process rather than foreclosed, and subjectivities are too complex, dynamic and non-essential to allow easy prediction of racialised identities from snapshots of children's lives. In addition, both social class and gender differentiate the racialised experiences of people of mixed parentage and of black people. For example, we found in this study that middle-class black and mixed-parentage young people are more likely than those from the working classes to live in neighbourhoods, and attend schools, that are almost exclusively white. As a result, their friends and the people they spend time with also tend to be white, with the result that they are not necessarily as comfortable or as familiar with black people as might be expected. These issues are discussed further in the chapters that follow.

3   Identity and mixed parentage

Theory, policy and research

In Chapter 2 we discussed what is known about attitudes in the past and currently to people of mixed parentage. As the proportion of the population who are of mixed parentage has increased, so more research and writing has been done on their own attitudes to their parentage, that is, to their racial identity. When the first edition of this book was published (in 1993), very little information on this topic was available – mainly only for eminent historical figures. Mary Seacole, for example, whose life we outlined in Chapter 2, described herself to her English readers as 'only a little brown – a few shades darker than the brunettes whom you admire so much' (Seacole, 1984: 58). But she was far from denying or despising her own ancestry. When an American admirer suggested that 'if we could bleach her by any means we would, and thus make her acceptable in any company, as she deserves to be', she retorted angrily:

> 'If it [her complexion] had been as dark as any nigger's, I should have been just as happy and as useful, and as much respected by those whose respect I value; and as to his offer of bleaching me, I should, even if it were practicable, decline it without any thanks. As to the society which the process might gain me admission into, all I can say is that judging from the specimens I have met with here and elsewhere, I don't think I shall lose much from being excluded from it.'

(Ibid.: 98)

Samuel Coleridge-Taylor, the composer, married a white English woman, and most of his friends were white. But not only did he turn to black folk music for much of his inspiration, he also involved himself in the political struggle of black people, and was elected to the executive committee of the newly formed Pan-African Association. Yet he remained very aware of his mixed parentage, and at the time of his death was working on an operetta about the intermarriage of white and black people (Sayers, 1915). On the other hand, the early nineteenth-century Jamaican-born revolutionary, William Davidson, identified strongly with the white English and their history, and appears to have denied that he had any association with black people (Mackey, 1972). And Thomas Freeman, the Methodist missionary, who was very light-skinned, felt himself to be both English and white and was so regarded by the Africans with whom he worked (Walker, 1929).

The marginal man

Racial identity became the subject of theorising by American sociologists from about 1930, although the term was not then in use. By this time anthropologists were arguing that differences between peoples are due to social processes, not innate racial differences, and biological explanations of human behaviour were beginning to lose their hold on academics, if not the general public. The intellectual climate was thus ripe for a discussion of the psychological and social implications of being of mixed parentage. Given the much larger size of the black population in the USA and the long-standing belief that people of mixed parentage were a problematic group, it is not surprising that the first social scientists to theorise about them were North Americans. There was another reason for their interest. Until the Second World War, sociologists in the USA were very concerned with their country's role as a 'melting-pot' for diverse cultures, and the difficulties to which this gave rise. They saw 'mulattos' as only one of many groups who experienced what would today be called identity problems.

The terms 'identity problems' and 'identity crisis' did not come into use until the 1950s, but in 1928 Robert Park, a Harvard sociologist, introduced the concept of 'the marginal man'. This described the predicament of those 'predestined to live in two cultures and two worlds', who inevitably experienced a divided self. However, while the marginal man was 'condemned by fate to live in two antagonistic cultures', Park stressed that this position brought great benefits. The marginal man can 'look with a certain degree of critical detachment' on both cultures, and is thus a citizen of the world. Inevitably, Park argued, his (*sic*) horizons are wider, his intelligence keener, his viewpoint more rational, than those of people who live within one culture (Park, 1928: 881).

Park went on to apply the concept to 'hybrid' people who live on the margin of two races. It is this position in society, and not heredity, that he believed 'makes the mulatto more intelligent, restless, aggressive and ambitious than the negro'. In support of this argument, he pointed out that the two most eminent American negro leaders, Booker T. Washington and W.E.B. du Bois, were both 'mixed-bloods' (Park, 1931: 534). Park's ideas were elaborated by a colleague, Everett Stonequist. Unlike Park, Stonequist saw little that was positive in the marginal situation. His major contributions were to analyse the psychological difficulties it created, and to add a developmental dimension. He argued that there is a life cycle in marginality. In the first phase of the cycle marginal individuals, such as 'half-castes' (as people of mixed black and white parentage were called by then), are not conscious or only dimly conscious, of their difference from the dominant caste. In the second phase a crisis occurs. Through some act of rejection they become aware that they are marginal; that is, that in the eyes of white people, with whom they are at least partially identified, they belong to an inferior and despised group.

This situation is inherently painful, and Stonequist believed that it is inevitably accompanied by psychological maladjustment. At its minimum this consists of a feeling of isolation, of not quite belonging anywhere, and, at its extreme, of feelings of despair. In the third stage of the cycle the half-castes attempt to escape from the painful state of marginality by 'adjustment'. They may decide to become fully absorbed in the white group by 'passing' as white, where this is a possibility. Or they may decide to become assimilated into the black group, although to do so they will have to overcome their negative feelings towards black people, and the distrust and hostility of black people towards themselves. Some may choose to remain marginal, forever condemned to feel isolated and rejected by both groups. This state is likely to lead to delinquency or despair, but a few individuals will be strong enough to live with their social isolation, and insist on their dual status in both groups, maintaining that 'I refuse to deny myself' (Stonequist, 1937: 138).

Stonequist's exposition of marginality echoes the theme of many US novels written from the late nineteenth century onwards. The stereotypical presentation by white authors involved a beautiful, upper-class, almost white heroine, often an 'octoroon' (i.e. with one black great-grandparent) who discovers as an adult that she has black ancestry. The discovery is shattering. Typically, the heroine loses her white lover and meets a tragic end. Rejected by the white community, resented and envied by the black community with whom she cannot identify and whom she despises, she is doomed to self-hatred (Berzon, 1978: 119–139).

Both black and white American novelists explored the ways in which this crisis can be resolved. The hero or heroine may decide to 'pass' as white, with all the attendant fear of exposure, and the guilt and self-hatred of denying family, friends and roots. In the black-authored books they are more likely to come to realise that happiness and self-esteem can only be found within the black community, by becoming leaders, or schoolteachers, or by serving it in other ways, or simply through acceptance of black values and a black way of life.

The theory of marginality is much more subtle and rich than it is often given credit for. It includes the notion of the 'outsider', who lives on the margins of two cultures or peoples, but it is quite distinct from the concept of alienation. Marginal individuals are not alienated, but on the contrary feel the pull of both cultures. They experience a divided self, because they internalise the attitudes of both groups to each other. The concept can be used to illuminate a variety of predicaments, for example, that of people whose education moves them from the working class to the middle class, but who thereafter never feel truly at ease with either class. (This situation is described by several authors in Heron, 1985.) Renamed 'between two cultures', the concept continued in widespread currency for a long time.

However, it is important to realise that the theory was not supported by any empirical investigations. It was presumably based on personal observations (supplemented, perhaps, by novel reading). One sociologist in the 1950s set out to test the theory by interviewing second-generation male American Jews whose parents had immigrated from Eastern Europe. He found that only a small minority experienced their situation as a conflict. An equal number had a positive 'dual orientation'. These men considered it unimportant whether or not people were Jewish; they associated with both Jews and non-Jews, choosing their friends on the basis of whether they liked them, and they expected that a slow and steady integration of Jews would occur. But the largest group, just over a half, lived within the Jewish community, feeling little pull towards non-Jewish American society. The author points out that although the *situation* of American Jews was marginal, as *individuals* the men he interviewed had worked out a variety of ways of life which were 'relatively smooth, liveable and satisfying' (Antonovsky, 1956). No such studies were made – in the United States or elsewhere – of racially mixed people. Nevertheless, the belief that they will almost inevitably experience a divided self, with consequent psychological problems, which are best solved by becoming full members of the black community, has been very widely accepted.

While it is well known that there has been strident opposition to 'racial mixing', it is possible to discern positive as well as negative themes in views on it over the past sixty years. As described above, in 1931, for example, the sociologist Robert Park argued that there could be positive benefits of the marginality resulting from mixed parentage, in that the possession of two cultures could make the marginal person a 'citizen of the world'. This conceptualisation of 'marginality' is, arguably, a forerunner of current notions of 'border crossing', which celebrate mixed parentage as allowing privileged access to a plurality of cultures and racialised groups (EYTARN, 1995). Root (1996) suggests that there are four ways in which biracial people negotiate their identities: having feet in both camps; practising situational ethnicity and situational race; sitting on the border, and using it as a central reference point; and situating oneself in one 'camp' for extended periods of time (but making occasional forays outside).

Research on the identity of children and adolescents of black and mixed parentage

The issue of how people of mixed parentage perceive themselves is nowadays couched in terms of identity, not marginality. The terms *identity*, *identity confusion*, *identity problems* and *identity crisis* have entered common usage, filtered through from the work of psychologists such as Erikson (1968). Erikson viewed adolescence as a stage in life when identity problems almost invariably occur. Young people, he believed, become very conscious at this time of the inconsistencies in their behaviour and values, and feel uncertain about what sort of person they are, and what they want to do with their lives. An adolescent with a mild identity problem wrote the following description of herself:

> I am a human being. I am a girl. I am an individual. I don't know who I am. I am a Pisces. I am a moody person. I am an indecisive person. I am an ambitious person. I am a very curious person. I am not an individual. I am a loner. I am an American (God help me). I am a democrat. I am a liberal person. I am a radical. I am a conservative. I am a pseudo-liberal. I am an atheist.
>
> (Montemayor and Eisen, 1977: 318)

According to Erikson, in the turmoil of their attempts to achieve an integrated identity, adolescents experience an identity crisis from which they emerge, very changed, as integrated adults.

Many psychologists challenged this view of adolescence, but the concepts of identity confusion and identity problems have been widely used in discussions of racial identity. Research began in the late 1940s, when two black American psychologists, the Clarks, used black and white dolls to explore young children's racial identifications. The basic findings were that by the age of 3 the black children could correctly select the dolls that 'looked like a white child and like a coloured child'. However, when asked 'Give me the nice doll' half chose the white doll, and when asked 'Give me the doll that looks bad', half chose the black doll. A cause of particular concern was that one third of the black children 'misidentified' themselves, choosing the white doll in response to the request 'Give me the doll that looks like you' (Clark and Clark, 1947). In contrast, white children overwhelmingly identified themselves as white and said they preferred the white doll. These findings were subsequently replicated by many other researchers in a number of countries.

The studies were interpreted as evidence that black children suffer from identity confusion and low self-esteem because they internalise white people's negative view of their race. They were used to argue for the desegregation of US schools in 1954, in the case of Brown against the Board of Education. During the 1970s, replications of the studies showed a sharp drop in the proportion of black children who were thought to misidentify themselves as white, and also in the proportion of those who said that they would prefer to be white (see e.g. Davey and Norburn, 1980; Milner, 1983). This change is usually thought to have been caused by shifts in black consciousness engendered by the Black Power and civil rights movements in the 1960s and 1970s. More recently, studies of children and young people in Britain and the USA found evidence of white children and young people wishing to be black. For example, Boulton and Smith (1992) found that one third of the sample of white British children aged 8–11 chose photographs of African Caribbean children as the ones 'they would most like to be'. The authors believed that the finding reflected the popularity of local black sportsmen. For teenagers, particularly young men, it is the attractiveness of British African Caribbean and African American youth styles that inspires some to want to be black (e.g. Back, 1996; Frosh *et al.*, 2001; Hewitt, 1986; Majors and Billson, 1992).

Early studies of children and young people of mixed parentage: disrupting common-sense understandings

It was, and perhaps still is, folk wisdom that mixed-parentage children are likely to suffer more severe identity problems than are black children. 'But what about the children?' is a frequent response to a mixed marriage or partnership. It was also the message of the 'marginality' theorists, and, as we saw in Chapter 2, of popular fiction. After all, as Stonequist pointed out, the children are liable to experience rejection by both black and white people, perhaps even from their own extended families. The 'divided self' of which he spoke may take the form of a conflict of loyalty in relation to their parents, and may lead to identity confusion, and, as well as the stigma of their own mixed appearance, there is the additional stigma of living in a mixed household.

Although relatively little research has been done on children of mixed parentage, the few studies available have generally found these gloomy expectations to be unfounded. For example, Bagley and Young (1979), in a British study of sixty-four mixed-parentage children aged 4–7 found high levels of self-esteem, and positive attitudes to both black and white people. Another British study casts doubt on the 'marginal' theory that mixed-parentage children are rejected by both black and white people. This was the first British study specifically to address the issue of identity in mixed-parentage children living with their own parents (Wilson, 1987). Her study of fifty-one 9-year-old British children with one white and one African or African Caribbean parent found little evidence of identity confusion. She presented the children with a variety of photographs of black, white and mixed-parentage children. The great majority of the children – over 80 per cent – selected a photograph of a mixed-parentage, rather than a black or white child, as the one most like themselves. When asked which of the children they would rather be, while half chose the photograph of a child like themselves, just over one third chose one of a lighter-skinned child. The proportion who by this criterion were satisfied with their own racial identity was in fact higher than in the studies of children with two black parents reported above. Putting together all her findings, Wilson concluded that 14 per cent of the mixed-parentage children had a white identity, 8 per cent a black, 20 per cent were inconsistent, while 59 per cent saw themselves as neither black nor white, but as brown, 'coloured', 'half-and-half' or 'half-caste'. This 'intermediate' identification was made most often by children living in multiracial areas, while the children with 'inconsistent identities', or who saw themselves as white, were more likely to live in mainly white areas.

Wilson's study suggested that up to the age of 9, at any rate, the majority of the mixed-parentage children did not suffer from identity problems; she found them to be happy and secure with an intermediate identity. Nor have children of mixed parentage been found to be shunned by other children. For example, Durojaiye (1970), in a survey of friendship choices in Manchester junior school children, found that children of mixed parentage were frequently chosen as friends by both black and white children, although their own preference was for other children of mixed parentage. The only studies to report serious person-ality and identity problems in mixed-parentage children are clinical studies; that is, studies of children who come to notice because of their problems, as opposed to children found through schools or community networks.

However, it must be said that few such studies have been carried out, and they are mostly of young children. Little is known about the iden-tity of mixed-parentage young people living with their parents, although according to Erikson's identity theory, this is the stage when identity problems are likely to be most acute.

More recent studies of mixed parentage

Bothland rather than eitherlor identities

Since the first edition of this book was published, there has been more research on mixed parentage. The resulting literature has become less problem-oriented, focused more on 'insider accounts' and presents more complex analyses that question the notion of stable, unchanging identities and racialisation, and recognise that gender and social class are all-important to the identities of people of mixed parentage (Kahn and Denmon, 1997). While some researchers continue to see 'biracial ethnic identity' as problematic (e.g. Herring, 1995), this is now much less common. Indeed, Korgen (1998) found that among her sample of forty US biracial adults, those born after 1965 tended to claim biracial identities, while those born before did not. This indicates that racialised identities are dynamic, changing over time. New theories of identities (discussed in Chapter 1) have influenced new ways of thinking about identities and, arguably, complement concepts of biraciality, multi-raciality, mixed parentage, etc. For example, Root (1992) suggests that social ambiguity, fluid identities, despite generally rigid racial boundar-ies, and being grounded in duality and multiplicity, are all ways in which biracial people view themselves as defined and united. These are also features of social constructionist theories of identities. To some extent then, the literature available has not only burgeoned, but has begun to address the sorts of issues raised in the first edition of this book (see chapters 5–10).

Negotiating socially constructed borders

Most studies that focus on insider accounts generally find that people of mixed parentage view themselves as neither black nor white. There. are now a variety of publications by people who are themselves 'insiders' to mixed parentage. For example, in a two-year ethnographic study in Bristol with sixteen women and nine men, most of whom had African or African Caribbean fathers and white European mothers, Jayne Ifekwunigwe (1999), herself of 'multiethnic origin', found that there was a tension between how her participants designated themselves and knowing that many people would expect them to call themselves 'black'. Ifekwunigwe argues that simply referring to someone with the complex histories of people in her study as 'black' reduces the complexities of family stories and identification. From a study of eight 'mixed-race Britons' (including some of Asian–white mixed parentage), Yasmine Khan (in prep.) also found that her participants had gone beyond thinking only in terms of black and white. Such studies present some of the complexities that James McBride (1998) documents in his US-based autobiographical work in which he pays tribute to what his white mother did for her mixed-parentage children.

'Insider research' demonstrates that including people in a category 'mixed parentage' (which many refer to in different terms) lumps together people who differ in many ways. This is sometimes also a feature of 'outsider research'. For example, Ilan Katz's (1996) British research included families from a range of different racialised and ethnicised groups (including 'Asian', white and black) and with children of different ages. While such research produces convincing evidence that people of mixed parentage differ in some ways from both sets of their parents, while experiencing racism, the possible conclusions are limited by the heterogeneity of the samples. Root (1996) argues that people of 'different mixtures' share enough common experiences for multiraciality to be considered a category. However, this does not mean that people who would be included in such a multiracial category should be seen as constituting one cultural group.

Diversity within people of mixed parentage is illustrated in a study of ninety-three 13–18-year-old young people equally divided into 'biracial', 'African American' and 'Caucasian'. Field (1996: 222) gave psychometric questionnaires and interviews to this sample and found that the 'biracial adolescents had self-concepts that were just as positive as their monoracial peers'. They were the most diverse group in terms of their participation in, and enjoyment of, white and/or black culture (which Field refers to as having a black, white or bicultural reference group). Those biracial young people who had white reference groups had greater difficulty in developing a positive self-concept than did black and biracial young people who had bicultural or black reference groups. Field suggests that it is not the colour of reference groups per se that is important, but that it was those who actively rejected black culture and internalised racism who were more likely to have less positive self-concepts.

Root (1998) studied twenty biracial sibling pairs in the USA aged between 18 and 40 years. All her participants indicated that they became aware of gender before they became aware of 'race' by 5 or 6 years of age, and the women reported that they were viewed as particularly sexy and exotic because of their colour and background in ways not reported by the men. Root found that siblings of 'mixed-race heritage' differ in their identifications depending on their experiences and possibly 'colour coding'.

Racialisation of mixed parentage

Williams (1996) found in her pilot study of twenty biracial US adults (ten African/European American and ten Asian/European American) that many experienced racialising interactions through which they learned about their racialised self in childhood. She argues that 'the question *What Are You?* that is so often asked of racially mixed people unveils the racial, social disorientation of the person asking the question as much as it potentially dislocates the person being asked. The racially mixed person may feel doubly *other*ed by such constant interrogation' (Williams, 1996: 203). Willliams' interviewees reported commonly experiencing crises in racial meaning through being asked the marginalising, exoticising and alienating question *What Are You?* They felt this bound biracial people together and fortified their sense of biraciality as they actively created new racialised meanings during interactions. This raises the question of when mixed-parentage children begin to experience the *What Are You?* question as common. These racialising moments may arise in other ways. In a study of adult biracial siblings in the USA, Root found that 'hazing' (being forced to prove oneself an authentic insider, mostly as African American) affected the process of racial identity development. Some of the people whom she interviewed were resentful at being forced to prove their authenticity in stereotypical ways in order not to be excluded.

Root (1998: 243) suggests that 'a combination of mixed parentage and phenotype and assertions of biracial heritage . . . and multiethnic identity . . . were associated with hazing', in that someone equally light-skinned with two African American parents is less likely to be subjected to the harshness of hazing. The issue of 'chromatism' or 'colourism' was discussed in Chapter 1 as paradoxically having gained both socioeconomic privileges and discrimination for 'light-skinned' black people (who historically included people of mixed parentage). Cunningham (1997) found that colourism was reported to have had a profound effect on the eleven 'light skin blacks' aged 21–59 in the USA whom she interviewed – all of whom had two parents who were African American. She found that several of them reported that their families contained people who ranged widely in colour. Many reported difficult experiences to do with colour during their adolescence because people seemed uncertain about who they were and because some of their own family members did not accept them. Cunningham argues that their sense of exclusion fractured the relationship between lighter and darker black people. Yet, because her participants often had to acknowledge 'race' by explaining themselves, their identities were threatened at the same time that they had freedom to 'pass' as white or not to 'pass'. Twine (1996) found, in a study of sixteen African-descent US women students who had been 'culturally constructed' as white in their child-hood, that some constructed for themselves a black or biracial identity when they became students. 'Passing' could therefore be a temporary phase – as dynamic a process as other aspects of racialisation. Shade of colour is by no means a complete explanation for why people of mixed parentage experience racism and exclusion. However, the findings from Cunningham's study of 'light skin blacks' underlines the fact that any-body who appears not to fit definitively into either a white or a black category is likely to experience challenge, questioning and resentment.

In a small-scale study of nine 5- to 16-year-old biracial children in the USA (Kerwin et al., 1993), half said that they had not specifically been asked by anyone about their background. However, the four oldest par-ticipants could recall occasions when people had attempted to pressure them into choosing one colour as their primary identification and some talked of informal segregation at school so that black and white chil-dren did not mix. Few of the children could remember a racialising moment when they first became aware of racial categories. Morrison (1995) studied the self-concept of biracial pre-school children by inter-viewing eleven of their mothers and giving nine 3- to 5-year-old biracial children a picture story test designed to assess their racial attitudes (the Preschool Racial Awareness Measure – PRAM II). Seven of the nine children gave responses which showed no racial bias, one showed a pro-white/anti-black bias and one a pro-black/anti-white bias.

Parental views and contributions

Luke and Luke (1998, 1999) conducted a study of forty-two sets of couples in 'mixed-race' marriages where one partner was 'Indo-Asian'. They found that interracial couples had to negotiate cultural expectations about weddings, family life, children and in-laws, rather than being able to take for granted that there are clear norms to follow. They, therefore, had to construct their hybrid, multiple identities in relation to the social contexts in which they were positioned. At the same time, racialising practices constructed them as 'Other'. This rare Australian study suggests the more general finding that parents from different racialised and ethnicised groupings may face difficulties in sorting out their household cultural practices in raising their mixed-parentage children.

White mothers may also face a variety of difficulties in rearing their mixed-parentage children. These range from being called racist names and/or being physically attacked by white people in the street, to being excluded by black family members (Alibhai-Brown and Montague, 1992; Twine, 2001). For this reason, Leicestershire Constabulary in Britain became one of the first police forces to recognise that 'racial incidents' can involve white 'victims' who are targeted because they live in 'mixed-race' families. Interracial relationships were identified as a factor in 46 per cent of those 'racial incidents' reported by white 'victims' and as a factor in 'racial incidents' for 15 per cent of all victims (Webb, 1998). Twine (a 'biracial' US researcher) conducted a study of white birth mothers of mixed-parentage children in the British Midlands (1999a, 1999b, 2001). She found that the mothers often reported that they were viewed by the black relatives of their children as having access to 'white privilege'. They reported that they often faced negative racialisation, and sometimes exclusion, from black family members who believe that they cannot properly empathise with their children because they have never experienced racism. Their fear that black people might reject their children led some to use intricate strategies to counter racism and diminish the perceived racial gap between themselves and their children. For some, this entailed ensuring that they lived in neighbourhoods with several other black families.

Kerwin *et al.*, (1993) conducted a small-scale US qualitative study of racialised identity in biracial children, that included some of their parents. They found that some parents were unhappy that they have to provide racial designations for their children (e.g. in the Census) and some considered it problematic that there are no adequate labels to describe their children. Where two parents were interviewed, they sometimes did not agree about how their children would refer to them-selves if asked. Many were concerned to prepare their children for meeting racial discrimination and some deliberately chose to live in multiracial rather than monoracial neighbourhoods in order to avoid racism. In another US study, Morrison (1995) found that nine of the eleven mothers (nine white and two black) of biracial children whom she studied felt that it was important for their children to make racial identifications that reflect their mixed parentage backgrounds. Seven chose the term 'biracial', one chose 'mixed' and one (a white mother) favoured 'black'. The other two eschewed notions that racial identifica-tion was important. Most attempted to promote their children's iden-tity development by trying to teach their children about both parents' cultures, buying white and black dolls, etc. From his intensive study of twenty-one US families, Rosenblatt (1999) argues that the challenges faced by multiracial families can be intense, caused by racism and pressures for their children to identify as monoracial once they go to school.

In conclusion

Much of the work published about mixed parentage is on the basis of very small, self-selected samples in the USA. For example, Bowles (1993) presents work on ten young adults of mixed black/white parent-age whom she worked with over thirty years of clinical practice. Richards (1995) interviewed twelve young people ranging in age from 12–30 years, some of whom had been adopted. Thus, although more studies are available than previously and they provide useful insights, there is still a great need for larger scale, in-depth studies of samples that come from a wide strata of society in Britain and other countries as well as the USA.

The area of mixed relationships and mixed parentage is one where demography and social definitions can clearly be seen to intersect. The increasing number of 'mixed', black–white unions and people of 'mixed parentage', particularly young people, has been partly responsible for the emergence of insider-defined 'mixed' categories. These challenge the treatment of black and white racialised categories as binary opposites and the 'one drop' thesis that anybody with black ancestry is necessar-ily, and only, black. It is now much more commonly recognised than previously that people of 'mixed parentage' largely do not suffer from racialised identity problems and that most identify themselves as 'mixed'. This has partly been made possible by new ways of thinking of identities – as fluid, multiple and dynamic – and racialisation. However, most experience racism (from outsiders, and sometimes from within their families). The chapters that follow indicate the issues faced by young people of mixed parentage and their families as they negotiate socially constructed racialised boundaries.

4   The 'transracial adoption'/
'same race' placement debate

Introduction

The issue of how mixed-parentage children are racialised is an important aspect of the debate about transracial adoption. The debate almost always involves the adoption by white parents of children from minority ethnic groups and is concerned with whether this practice is legitimate, or whether only 'same-race' placements should be allowed. There has been considerable confusion about what is meant by 'same race', especially in the case of mixed-parentage children, unsurprisingly, since there is still widespread confusion and debate about how best to view and treat people of mixed parentage.

Transracial adoption was a rarity in Britain until the 1960s. During this decade, adoption, previously much stigmatised, became an increasingly acceptable way for some white couples to enlarge their family or solve the problem of infertility, and the number of adoption orders steadily increased. At first, children from minority ethnic groups were classed with those who had physical imperfections or questionable family histories as 'unadoptable'. However, by the mid-1960s the increase in the number of couples wishing to adopt led to a reconsideration of this attitude, and the British Adoption Project was initiated to answer the question 'Can families be found for coloured children?' By the end of the decade a combination of the Abortion Act of 1968, the increased assistance available for single mothers, and changing attitudes to 'illegitimacy' resulted in a sharp decline in the number of healthy able-bodied white babies placed for adoption. At the same time, the number of white couples seeking to adopt continued to grow. Since no effort was made to find black adoptive parents, who were thought unlikely to meet the criteria then considered necessary (for example, a married couple in comfortable housing with a good, steady income where the wife was not working), 'transracial adoptions' became increasingly common.

In the USA a similar trend was fiercely attacked by the National Association of Black Social Workers as early as 1972. A decade later the first major British attack took place, at the inaugural meeting of the Association of Black Social Workers and Allied Professions in 1983. As well as political reasons for this opposition, psychological reasons were also put forward. It was argued that:

- Unless they are very carefully trained, white families cannot provide black children with the skills and 'survival techniques' they need for coping in a racist society (Small, 1986).
- Black children growing up in white families fail to develop a positive black identity. Instead, they suffer identity confusion and develop a negative self-concept, believing or wishing that they were white, and harbouring negative attitudes towards black people (Maxime, 1986).
- In consequence their self-esteem is low, and their mental health damaged (Small, 1986).
- They will not only be rejected by white people, but also by black people, for not being 'black enough in culture and attitude' (Small, 1986; 92).

It was further argued that no distinction should be made between children with one or two black parents. According to one leading UK black social worker, John Small (1986: 91), the term 'mixed race' can lead to the belief that

> such children are racially distinct from other blacks. . . . Many black people find the term derogatory and racist because they feel it is a conscious and hypocritical way of denying the reality of a child's blackness. Certainly, mixed-race children are regarded as black by society and eventually the majority of such children will identify with blacks, except in instances where reality and self-image have not merged.

Small went on to argue that the term 'mixed race' is in any case inappropriate, because a majority of African Caribbeans have some white ancestors, and differ from 'mixed-race' children only in the time at which the mixture occurred.

Black social workers' critique of the concept of 'mixed race' and concern about the identities of children of 'mixed race' was made in the context of their opposition to the transracial adoption and fostering both of children of mixed parentage and those with two black parents.

In both the UK and the USA this opposition was grounded in the undoubted racism of some social work departments, where little or no effort was made to recruit black foster and adoptive parents, who were seen as unlikely to provide an adequate standard of care. Moreover, the importance of feeling positive about their 'race' was not taken into account when considering children's needs, so that they were sometimes placed with racist families. From the USA, Babb and Laws (2001) suggest that the one-way adoption of minority ethnic children by white parents partly results from racism:

> This one-way transracial adoption exists partly because a disproportionately high number of minority race children are waiting to be adopted. However, racism is also undoubtedly to blame for the lack of transracial adoptions involving the adoption of Caucasian children by minority race parents. Some of the same agency workers who allow Caucasians to adopt children of color hesitate to allow Caucasian children to be adopted into minority communities by adults of color.

In the 1980s, Small (a black UK social worker) and Maxime (a black UK psychologist) cited two kinds of evidence in support of an argument for 'same-race' placements. The first comes from case studies of disturbed black and mixed-parentage children in the care of white residential care staff or foster parents. One child, for example,

> came into care at 2 years and 9 months. He spent two subsequent years in a nursery. He was then placed with white foster parents and then placed for adoption with a white family because it was said there were no black families who would adopt him. The placement broke down because the father could not relate to a black child as his own. The boy at an earlier stage showed signs of 'identity confusion' by trying to scratch off his skin in the bath. He was placed with another family at the age of 9 years. He had said that he did not want a black family. The family had difficulties in caring for a black child. The placement broke down when Trevor was 13 years old. It was later discovered that he thought he was white. At 14 years old, it was discovered that he could not relate to black people. He also felt rejected by white society. His confusion manifested itself in conduct disorder. It was so severe that he was recommended for psychiatric treatment. He was eventually diagnosed a 'schizophrenic'.

(Small, 1984: 136)

This distressing account certainly suggests that white foster parents who cannot accept a black child may cause psychological damage. But we need to know how often damage of this kind occurs in black children placed with white families, and the contribution made to this boy's problems by a series of disrupted placements, which he experienced as rejections because of his colour. Unfortunately, very high rates of psychological disturbance and feelings of rejection occur among both black and white children in care. But if behaviour of this kind is not found among the majority of 'transracially adopted' children it would suggest that being cared for by white people does not in itself cause psychological problems and identity confusion.

Two studies, one British (Gill and Jackson, 1983) and one from the USA (Simon and Alstein, 1987), followed 'transracially adopted' children through their childhood to their early or mid-teens. Several other US studies, (Feigelman and Silverman, 1983; Grow and Shapiro, 1974; Kim *et al.*, 1979) have assessed them at one particular age. There are also a number of European studies of 'transracially adopted' children, mainly brought from South Asia and Latin America (see Tizard, 1991). With one exception, a study of the adoption of native Canadian children by white Canadians (Bagley, 1990), all studies of 'transracial adoption' have shown that black and mixed-parentage children who are adopted by white parents tend to have at least as high a level of self-esteem as white adopted children, that they tend to do as well at school, to have as good relations with their adoptive parents and with their peers, and to have no more behaviour problems than do white adopted children. This evidence would appear to refute the suggestion that black children reared by white parents will have low self-esteem and suffer from emotional disturbance.

However, the second line of evidence to which Small and his colleagues pointed in their attack on 'transracial adoption' is that the children in these studies have not developed a black identity. In a British study of 'transracial adoption', Gill and Jackson (1983) conducted a study of over thirty 13- to 15-year-olds who had been 'transracially adopted', and were from a wide range of ethnic groups, many of mixed parentage. They found that, on the whole, the young people were 'psychologically well-adjusted' with high self-esteem, happy in their families and doing well at school. However, when they were asked 'Which of the following statements fits how you really feel? A. I am proud to be coloured/black/brown; B. I don't really mind what colour I am; C. I would prefer to be white', only 14 per cent said they felt proud of their colour. Twenty per cent said they would rather be white, while the rest said they did not mind what colour they were. None of the children described themselves as black, but equally none described themselves as white; most said they were 'brown' or 'coloured'. In reply to a further question about whether, when they left home, they would like to spend more time with West Indian/Asian people, only 30 per cent said they would. Growing up in middle-class homes, they did not, for the most part, identify with the working-class black or Asian people they had seen on visits to the nearest city. Rather, they felt very distant from black people and said they had little in common with them. It is, of course, possible that their identifications may change in the future (Cunningham, 1997; Mama, 1995; Root, 1996).

Rather similar findings emerged from a US study (McRoy and Zurcher, 1983) which provided a particularly good test of Small's case, since it compared two groups of black and mixed-parentage adolescents, one adopted by white parents and another by black parents. The two groups of adolescents were generally well matched, but more of those adopted by white parents were of mixed parentage. Both sets of parents and children were said to have equally loving relationships, and none of the children felt they were 'outsiders' in the family. There was no difference in the self-esteem of the two groups of young people, and both groups were said to be strongly supported by their adoptive families and extended kin. This support 'overcame any negative labelling linked with being adopted or black' (McRoy and Zurcher, 1983: 123).

There was, however, a difference in the racialised identities of the two groups. The black adolescents adopted by white parents were more likely to have white friends and 'dates', and were more likely to refer to themselves as 'mixed' or 'part white', rather than black, or else to dismiss the importance of 'racial identity' by preferring to label themselves as a 'human being'. They were more likely to consider themselves dissimilar to other black people.

In the USA, Simon and Alstein have now followed up an initial sample of 204 3- to 7-year-old 'transracially adopted' children into adulthood (Simon, 1994; Simon and Alstein, 1977, 1981, 1987, 1996, 2000; Simon et al., 1994). At the second contact, when the children were aged between 11 and 15 years of age, they found that one in six of the parents whom they interviewed reported that their children were showing problems that they considered to be related to the 'transracial adoption'. However, at the end of the study, most parents (over 90 per cent) reported that they would 'do the same again'. Overall, the researchers did not find evidence of problems with racial identity in the 'transracially adopted' children. In their 1987 publication, they reported that 'transracially adopted' adolescents did not differ from white adoptees in self-esteem or the extent to which they were integrated into the family. Only 11 per cent said they would prefer to be white.

Several studies, therefore, provide evidence that black and mixed-parentage adolescents growing up in adopted white families do not generally believe that they are, or wish to be, white. They do, however, suggest that these young people will tend not to feel proud of their origin. To many white people pride in one's colour or ethnicity might seem unimportant, or even undesirable, but in the context of a racist society, feeling proud of being black is not analogous to feeling proud of being white. If the majority stigmatise one's colour, then to be proud of it is likely to be a protective factor. The studies also suggest that these young people will not think of, or label themselves, as black. However, it should be noted that a substantial proportion of the young people in these studies were of mixed parentage. This was the case with just under half of the children in the US longitudinal study (Simon and Alstein, 1981: 13). In the case of the British study, almost half had a white mother, only one-fifth had one or two African or African Caribbean parents, while the majority had Asian or Anglo-Asian backgrounds. There is some evidence to suggest that if they had been living with their families of origin most may well not have called themselves black (see Modood, 1988; Wilson, 1987). And, as we have shown, the evidence available does not support the view that calling themselves 'brown', rather than 'black' has implications for their mental health.

As for the tendency for the 'transracially adopted' adolescents to have mainly white friends, it should be remembered that the majority of the young people in both the British and US studies lived in predominantly white communities, and attended schools where there were very few, if any, other black children. According to the USA researchers McRoy and Zurcher, 'the opportunity for establishing positive relationships with blacks on an everyday basis was a key factor in the child's development of a positive black identity and a corresponding feeling about other blacks' (1983: 134). They found that black adolescents adopted by white parents who lived in 'racially' mixed communities, attended 'racially' integrated schools, and who had parents who regarded the children as black, rather than 'mixed' tended to think positively about themselves as black.

The evidence reviewed above therefore suggests that 'transracially adopted' children are likely to have as high a self-esteem, to be as closely attached to their parents, to do as well at school, and to have no more psychological problems than other adopted children. If they are of mixed parentage or Asian, they are likely to think of themselves as 'mixed' or 'brown', rather than 'black'. If they live in a multiracial community, and thus have the opportunity, they are likely to have black friends and to think positively about their colour.

Over the past few years, however, critiques of studies producing such conclusions have begun to emerge. Various reviews now point to methodological flaws in many studies that have shown no deleterious effects of 'transracial adoption'. For example, Alexander and Curtis (1996) argue that the reliance on qualitative studies or those using low-level statistics and no comparison groups make less definite conclusions than has been assumed. They argue that 'these shortcomings aside, certainly, the weight of the research evidence favours proponents of 'transracial adoption', albeit all the evidence was not produced by the strongest research methodology' (p. 231). Hollingsworth (1997) conducted a meta-analytic review of studies on 'transracial adoption' (which aggregates the samples of similar studies in order to produce more clear-cut findings than is possible from one study). She found that these analyses raised questions about the 'racial identity' of 'transracially adopted' children, but not about their self-esteem. However, there were only six studies that did not suffer from problems such as data being collected only from adoptive parents, rather than adoptees themselves, or that did not omit 'same-race' placements. For these reasons, only six studies met her criteria for inclusion in her meta-analysis. Hollingsworth concludes that continued careful study is needed to tell us what are the best interests of children to be adopted. She also identifies ignorance about the effects of 'transracial adoption' on biracial children. Similarly, Park and Green (2000) argue that not only methodological difficulties, but also ethnocentrism in research studies, leave open the question of how 'transracial adoption' affects black and other minority ethnic children.

To these criticisms must be added the problem of using longitudinal studies (valuable as they often are) to decide current policy, since the longitudinal studies cited above mostly concerned children adopted in infancy or as toddlers. Nowadays, however, children are rarely placed in infancy and are more likely to have complex psychological issues to deal with. In addition, because 'open adoption' is now the standard, they may well retain links with their birth parents. Such changes unfortunately limit the relevance of earlier studies on 'transracial adoption'.

The 'transracial adoption'/'same-race' placement controversy

Regardless of the research findings available at the time, in the USA a national policy of 'same-race' adoption was pursued and 'transracial' placements dropped dramatically (Hayes, 1993). In Britain, according to Rhodes (1992: 202), most local authorities had adopted the principle of 'racial matching' by the end of the 1980s, which involved placing children of mixed parentage only with black or racially mixed couples. Racial factors were given official recognition in the Children Act 1989, which stated that 'In making any such decision a local authority shall give due consideration. . . to the child's religious persuasion, racial origin and cultural and linguistic background'. This statement allows for a wide variety of interpretations, but the policy guidelines issued from the Social Services Inspectorate (Utting, 1990: 3), while leaving open the possibility of 'transracial' placement in exceptional circumstances, stated that 'other things being equal and in the great majority of cases, placement with a family of similar ethnic origin and religion is most likely to meet a child's needs'.

Nonetheless, the 'transracial adoption'/'same-race' placement controversy continued to rage at the end of the twentieth century and remains an issue at the beginning of the twenty-first. Because it has been very heated and has clearly not been settled by research evidence, it is important to take a close look at the arguments put forward in order to understand why controversy has been so long-lasting and passionate.

The debate is usually seen as having polarised 'sides' ('for' and 'against'). The controversy centres on the issue of whether the placement of black children and those from other minority ethnic groups with white foster or adoptive parents damages the 'racial identities' of the children. Proponents of 'transracial adoption' do not necessarily disagree that black and other minority ethnic children should ideally go to black and minority ethnic group parents, a position endorsed by the Children Act 1989 (e.g. Gaber and Aldridge, 1994). They are, thus, not always on opposite sides from proponents of 'same-race' placements. However, they argue that black children's interests are better served by placement in loving white majority ethnic homes that provide continuity of care, rather than in institutions or multiple placements.

Both sides of this debate draw on arguments about children's psychosocial development and, as discussed above, to some extent both find support from the few studies that have been carried out on 'transracial adoption'. As we have seen, there is some clinical evidence that a few transracially adopted children do suffer severe problems of identity (Maxime, 1986; Small, 1986). However, while clinical evidence is important, it is not sufficient to the task of providing support for one or other side of the debate since it is not possible to generalise from small numbers of exceptional cases. Furthermore, there is also clinical evidence that a small percentage of black children and children of mixed parentage living with their birth parents also experience severe identity problems (e.g. Banks, 1992, 1996, 1999).

How then is it possible to make sense of the polarised impasse in this controversy? The discussion below teases apart the issues raised by strong versions of both positions to demonstrate that such complex questions are not adequately dealt with from entrenched, opposed, positions. It is worth noting that none of the positions discussed below differentiates black children from children of mixed parentage. However, it is increasingly being recognised that some children of mixed parentage live only with a white parent (Banks, 1995; Barn, 1993), and that it is therefore not justifiable to treat them as if they were identical to black children.

Positions which support 'transracial adoption'

It is clearly important for children to be brought up in households where they are loved, considered important and given continuity of care. However, the construction of a stark opposition between 'pro-' and 'anti-' 'transracial adoption' positions generally precludes recognition that this one psychological position (that children need love and continuity of care) includes people who have different political and psychological perspectives. Thus, there are five overlapping positions that those who are 'pro-transracial adoption' may support:

1 'Love is all you need'

If continuous love and care from one or two parent figures is sufficient to override all other considerations in childcare, the implication is that there is a hierarchy of children's psychological needs, with loving nurturance in a family being at the top. Few people would wish to deny the importance of loving, continuous care. However, more work is needed on the place of 'race' in children's lives in racialised societies. Clearly it is unsatisfactory to place black children, and those from other minority ethnic groups, with adults who do not recognise that they will face racism and who are determined to ignore the colour and ethnicity of children in their care.

2 Colour-blindness and the denial of racism

The extreme version of the 'colour-blind' argument, that colour plays little or no part in northern societies and is therefore irrelevant to children's lives, is extremely easy to refute and is not often presented.

Demographic data illustrate that there are continuing racialised inequities in many countries (see, e.g. Owen, 1994), while various studies (in psychology and other disciplines) illustrate the ways in which racism continues to operate (Commission for Racial Equality, 1985, 1988). Many people persist in arguing that young children are not yet racialised and do not notice 'race'. However, there is much evidence to the contrary which ranges from the work of the black psychologists Kenneth and Mamie Clark in the 1930s through to more recent research (e.g. Holmes, 1995; Troyna and Hatcher, 1992; Wright, 1992). For example, Ogilvy *et al.* (1990, 1992) found that nursery teachers treat, and respond differently to, Asian Scottish children than they do to white Scottish children, while James (1997) found that white London primary school children in ethnically mixed schools produce negative, racialised discourses of Asian people.

Paradoxically, a less extreme version of the 'return to colour-blindness' argument raises more serious and insidious issues which require the political motivation for denials of racism to be questioned. In Britain, as in various other countries, many black people and some white people have struggled to document and change some of the injustices of racism. Groups of black social workers have done much within their profession to put racism on the social work agenda. In the area of 'same-race' placement they have had a marked impact, even if they remain in professionally precarious positions (Lewis, 2000). In particular, the adoption of 'same-race' placement policies by many social work departments was in recognition of the prevalence of racism and its deleterious consequences. The late 1980s and 1990s, however, have been characterised by a retreat from engagement with issues of racism in the USA and in Britain. The term 'political correctness' has been used as an insult to defuse opposition to racism, sexism and hetero-sexism. In this context, some of those who attack political correctness welcome challenges to 'same-race' placement policies. In treating racism as non-existent, 'colour-blind' practices help to disempower black social workers (and black clients and potential parents) by treating their concerns about racism as irrelevant. Since black social workers are treated as problematic in many social work departments (Lewis, 1996), colour-blind approaches also deny the existence of racisms within the social work profession.

3 The success of 'transracial adoption'

Many proponents of 'transracial adoption' point to its success in turning out happy and successful adults. Those who have found in their research that 'transracial adoption' does not seem to damage the racialised identities of black children are particularly clear that 'transracial adoption' has been so successful that it should not be debarred (Simon 1994; Simon and Alstein, 1977, 1981, 1987; Simon *et al.*, 1994) – especially if parents live in 'racially heterogeneous settings' (Feigelman, 2000).

For a very few academics, it is a short step from arguing that 'transracial adoption' has been successful, to arguing that it is advantageous for black children to be reared in white, middle-class homes. Here, as in the issue of 'colour-blindness' and denial of racism (discussed above), the implications of research findings are given a particular slant, without acknowledgement of political bias. In the early 1980s, for example, Sandra Scarr engaged in debate with psychologists, social scientists and geneticists about transracial adoption. This followed from the publication of a paper by Scarr and Weinberg (1976) which suggested that it was parenting from white people, rather than economic advantage, that was responsible for 'the above-average IQ scores of black/interracial children adopted transracially'. Arguments about the biases in IQ tests have long been presented (Henwood and Phoenix, 1996). Yet, in Scarr and Weinberg's argument, 'transracial adoption' is constructed as providing a compensatory environment for black children. Not surprisingly, this publication generated a great deal of controversy, with Oden and MacDonald (1983) suggesting that the social commentary concluding the article made it unsuitable for publication.

This questionable position, of advocating 'transracial adoption' as a compensatory environment, is rarely voiced. However, it does surface from time to time. For example, Bartholet (1994:168) suggests that 'whites are in the best position to teach black children how to manoeuvre in the white worlds of power and privilege', while implying that some of the black adopters who have been recruited in recent years are not up to the task of childrearing. Arguably, while demonstrated success does not warrant legislation against transracial adoption, it does not justify encouraging 'transracial adoption'. The differential positioning of black and white people, and the economic resources available to them, continue to be important considerations. As with the wording of the Children Act, then, the argument that 'transracial adoption' is successful for most children who experience it leaves open, rather than either supporting or opposing, its practice.

4 Impracticality of a ban

The argument that a ban on 'transracial adoption' is unrealistic (and unkind) arises from the continued reported lack of black and minority ethnic group families willing to adopt children. However, it is difficult to establish how many black children and those from other minority ethnic groups are waiting to be placed at any one time:

> The fact that this information is still so hard to procure, despite being of major public importance, is perhaps due to the low priority it has been afforded or to its sensitive nature: such figures are notoriously difficult to collate due to the difficulties in agreeing on definitions of ethnicity and the precise meaning of 'waiting for placement'.
>
> (Rushton and Minnis, 1997:156)

If scarcity of black adopters is the only reason for allowing 'transracial adoption', extensive efforts, like those of some social services departments, should be made to remedy the situation. Unfortunately, social services commitment to increase the number of black adoptive and foster parents has, at least in the past, sometimes been more rhetorical than actual. In her study of foster care placements in one London borough, Rhodes (1992: 257) found that:

> Within the borough of the case study, the apparent radicalism and rapid pace of change belied an inherent conservatism which began to reassert itself as the immediate pressure to recruit black foster parents declined. The emphasis on team consensus and strategies of conflict avoidance prevented serious challenge to the status quo. The fragility of the new moves rapidly became obvious as the more radical initiatives, one by one, were dropped and the Fostering Team reverted to its old practices and approach. . . . What had, only weeks earlier, been declared 'top priority' was overtaken by 'more pressing needs' – a shortage of white foster parents. The excuse of resource constraints allowed the Team to continue to pay lip service to the goal of same 'race' placement whilst withdrawing from any practical commitment.

It is clear that many local authorities do make a lot of effort to recruit black foster and adoptive parents. However, as Rushton and Minnis (1997) argued, data on such issues continue to be surprisingly scarce at the beginning of the twenty-first century.

5 'Race' and ethnicity should not be theorised in essentialist and static ways

Some of those who are in favour of 'transracial adoption' base their support on the theorising of 'race' and ethnicity which is informed by postmodernism and critiques of essentialism. From such a position they argue that people in the same racialised groups may well have different identities and that these identities are not fixed, but may change over time. Furthermore, there are similarities between those in different racialised groups. They thus challenge the essentialist notions of identity used in some 'anti-transracial adoption' arguments. Table 4.1 summarises the implications of particular 'pro-transracial adoption' positions for social work practice.

Table 4.1: Implications of type of 'pro-transracial adoption' position for social work practice

Type of 'pro-transracial adoption' position	Implication for social work practice
Love overrides all other concerns with respect to children's needs and childcare	Little attention should be paid to 'race' or ethnicity in the placement of children
Social work practice should return to 'colour-blind' policies	The existence of racism is denied, so no account should be taken of 'race' or ethnicity
'Transracial adoption' is successful in producing children who fare well	Attention may or may not be paid to 'race', but 'transracial adoption' should be allowed. In its extreme version, 'transracial adoption' would be preferred
The impracticality of a blanket ban on transracial adoption	Racism and ethnicity are both taken into account but 'transracial' placements are made if 'same-race' placements are not available; what is meant by 'not available' is open to question
'Race' and ethnicity should not be theorised in essentialist and static ways	'Race' and racism are taken seriously, but 'transracial adoption' is not banned

Positions which oppose 'transracial adoption'

Just as those who support 'transracial adoption' may have different reasons for supporting it, so too opponents of 'transracial adoption' come from different positions. There are four main perspectives that are commonly expressed from the 'anti-transracial adoption' viewpoint. These partially intersect.

1 The politically indefensible 'stealing of children'

In the 1980s, David Devine (then Assistant Director of social services in Camden, later Assistant Director of CCETSW) made many media appearances in which he argued that 'transracial adoption' constituted the 'stealing of children' from the black community. It was, therefore, the supreme demonstration of the use of power by white society against black people. He frequently drew on his experience of having been 'transracially adopted' to argue against the policy. The limitations of using personal experience as the basis on which to draw policy conclusions was demonstrated in those programmes since Devine was often faced by Ben Brown, also a senior social worker who had been 'transracially adopted' and who was in favour of the continuation of the practice.

In considering Devine's argument, it is important to remember that black children who are 'looked after' by local authorities will not necessarily be fostered in black families, or cared for by black residential childcare workers if they are not 'transracially adopted'. Instead, black children often stay in care with a variety of white carers. For this reason, some of those who are against 'transracial adoption' as politically indefensible accept that, in keeping with current legislation, it may have to be used as a default position if permanent black carers are not quickly found (just as some of those who are in favour of 'transracial adoption' accept that it should only be a default position).

2 Racism overrides all

This position intersects with all the other positions in the 'anti-transracial adoption' argument, although the other positions do not necessarily entail the 'racism overrides all' position. Basically, the argument is that racism is so damaging to black children that black children should only live with black parents who have experienced racism and who can help these children to understand and deal with it. It thus employs the essentialist notion that all black parents will be able to help their children to deal with racism, while also assuming that white parents will not be able to help their children to understand, or to deal with, racism.

3   *Racialised and ethnicised separatism*

The notion that different 'races' and ethnic groups should not mix is a well-worn argument that is more usually held by white supremacists. However, more recently, black nationalists have responded to continuing outrages of racism by arguing that black people should keep themselves as far apart from white people as possible. Since 'transracial adoption' necessarily involves contact (although not sexual) between black and white people, these two politically divergent positions are united in the 'transracial adoption' controversy. People who are adamantly opposed to racism can thus espouse the same practices as those who are its most vociferous supporters. Gilroy (1996:72) argues that 'enemies' ('white supremacists and black absolutists, klansmen and black nationalists, zionists and anti-semites') can understand the world in the same way and, hence, can be political allies.

The separatist position is arguably as indefensible as the suggestion (e.g. from Bartholet, 1994) that 'transracial adoption' promotes 'racial integration' through mixing. The futility of this argument is demonstrated by, for example, the fact that heterosexual marriage between two consenting adults has not produced gender equity.

4   *'Transracial adoption' produces 'identity confusion'*

Perhaps the most rehearsed argument against 'transracial adoption' is that it damages the racial identity of black children and those from other minority ethnic groups (discussed above). According to this argument, black or mixed-parentage children brought up in white households may develop well in some ways, but will suffer from 'identity confusion', fail to develop a 'positive black identity' and be unable to relate to other black people. Furthermore, unless they are very well trained, white parents will be unable to pass on to black children the strategies they need in order to survive in a society where racism is common and where some degree of rejection by white people is likely (Maxime, 1986; Small, 1986). Since it is possible, in this argument, for white parents to be well trained so that they can pass on strategies for surviving racism, this position opens up the possibility that, if there are no other options, some white parents might be allowed to adopt black children (Table 4.2).

Table 4.2: Implications of 'anti-transracial adoption' position for social work practice

Type of 'anti-transracial adoption' position	Implications for social work practice
The politically indefensible 'stealing of children'	'Transracial adoption' allowed as a last resort, default position
Racism overrides all	'Transracial adoption' not allowed under any circumstances
Racialised and ethnicised separatism	'Transracial adoption' not allowed under any circumstances
'Transracial adoption' produces 'identity confusion'	'Transracial adoption' allowed as a last resort, provided that white parents are well trained about racism.

Contributions from research on racialisation and identity

Research cannot claim to be able to resolve the 'transracial adoption' debate. However, in conjunction with research from other disciplines and by making explicit the political arguments, it can be used to move it forward. Since psychological work can be used to support both sides of the debate, there is a need to conceptualise 'transracial adoption' in ways that do not reproduce the current oppositions. Instead, the complexities that are part of the racialisation of childhood need to be considered when making decisions about 'looked after' children.

Racism and racialisation are always part of black, mixed-parentage and other minority ethnic group children's lives

Although some proponents of the 'transracial adoption' position would like to take a 'colour-blind' approach, there has, for a long time, been a wealth of evidence which indicates that the lives of very young children are racialised (e.g. Clark and Clark, 1939, 1947; Holmes, 1995). To take a 'colour-blind' approach is thus to ignore the evidence that exists. In addition, it reproduces societal power relations by leaving the racialisation of white children from the majority ethnic group unquestioned and denying the experiences of racism faced by black and other minority ethnic group children. This can have deleterious effects on black children and those from other minority ethnic groups. In the first of her 1997 Reith lectures, Patricia Williams, a black professor of law in the USA, made this abundantly clear with an evocative example. When her son was aged 3, his nursery teacher told her that he seemed to be colour-blind. It turned out, however, that it was not that he could not distinguish colours but that, when asked to name a colour, he would reply 'it doesn't matter'. This, it turned out, was because his friends at nursery school had told him that he could not be a superhero, since superheroes could not be black. In response to his distress about this, the teacher had told him that colour 'doesn't matter'. The well-meaning teacher had, with one small comment, negated the pain of this child's experience, produced an unintended educational problem for him and left his white friends sanguine in their racialised beliefs. This example provides insight into why a 'colour-blind' approach is not tenable in the 'transracial adoption' debate.

Opponents of 'transracial adoption' construct it as the prime site of problems for black children. However, the psychological evidence indicates that this is not the case. The data that exist on 'racial identities' suggest that the process of identity development is difficult and painful for many non-adopted young black children (Hutnik, 1991; Milner, 1983). Yet, the self-esteem of young black people is not discernibly different from that of young white people (Phinney and Rosenthal, 1992; Phinney *et al.*, 1990; Spencer, 1990). These data suggest that learning to recognise and deal with racism may well be a painful process for many black children.

The theorisation of racialised identities: blackness as dynamic, plural and contested

An important point at issue between 'pro-' and 'anti-' groups relates to theories of identities. This is rarely the focus of discussion. Yet, it is a key area in which psychology can provide insights that may inform the debate. At the heart of the notion of black, 'transracially adopted' children developing 'a positive black identity' is the idea that there is one identity position which black people should occupy. Self-esteem and self-concepts are considered to be necessarily interlinked with black identity in one-to-one correspondence. This notion dates back to early work on racial identity which assumed that black children who 'misidentified' themselves as white would suffer from 'identity confusion' which would adversely affect them and their educational attainment. This argument was central to the 1954 Brown vs. the Board of Education desegregation case, which initiated the process of desegregation of schools in the USA (Clark, 1963). The Clarks' research (1939, 1947) was the single most quoted piece of research in this case, with a central argument being that school segregation damaged the racial identities of black children.

The interpretation of these data has been disputed, since there was no evidence that the deleterious effects of segregation on black children were linked to the racial segregation of schools (Murphy *et al.*, 1983). However, similar assumptions about self-esteem and positive black identity continue to be made (Katz, 1995). In recent decades, it has been shown that some young white people sometimes wish to be black (Hewitt, 1986; Jones, 1988). However, this has not been similarly interpreted as evidence of psychological pathology, probably because it is taken for granted that it is young black, not white, people who are likely to suffer from identity problems.

The idea that 'transracial adoption' impairs the development of a 'positive black identity' suggests there is a single way in which black identity can be positive. Yet the very notion of what it means to be black is dynamic, shifting with changes in political agenda and social theory (Gilroy, 1994). While the political and psychological are interlinked, it would seem to make more sense to think of black identities as plural and changing, rather than as unitary and static. Furthermore, the term 'black' constitutes part of a contested terrain, since part of the reason for its shifts in meaning is that some of those included and some of those excluded from it continually campaign (in various ways) to change its usage. In addition, identities also change over time, so that a younger black or mixed-parentage child who wants to be white may change her/his view as a teenager because of experiences at school, university or in employment. Mama (1995) found that the black women she interviewed reported such changes, as did the 'light-skinned' women interviewed by Cunningham (1997), who said they began to identify as black once they went to university.

It continues to be common for psychological work to simplify the notion of ethnic identity – despite the more complex psychological theorising of social identities discussed in Chapter 1. Much psychological work on 'ethnic identity' and 'racial identity' assumes that, for members of minority ethnic groups, ethnic identity is of central importance and must, essentially, be positive (Phinney and Rosenthal, 1992). Indeed, Phinney *et al.* (1990) suggest that minority ethnic group members will suffer confusion and despair if they fail to achieve an ethnic identity. Such work misses the fact that ethnic identity is plural, so that there are a variety of ways in which it may be experienced and may intersect with other identities. It also ignores the importance of ethnic identity to majority ethnic groups, probably because this is often not recognised (e.g. Cohen, 1988; Fine *et al.*, 1997; Frankenberg, 1993a,

1993b). Yet we know that, where young people from the majority ethnic group feel themselves to be lacking an ethnic identity, there can be dangerous tensions between them and those from minority ethnic groups (Macdonald *et al.*, 1989). Research on ethnic identity therefore lends support to the idea that 'ethnic identity' should be a major consideration in social work decisions about children from minority ethnic groups.

The essentialist view, of a one-to-one correspondence between a 'positive black identity' and self-esteem, is not supported by research evidence. From a review of mainly US work, Jackson *et al.* (1986: 248) argue that there has been a simplistic assumption that self-esteem and black identity are necessarily related, although 'empirical evidence to support this self-evident assumption is lacking'. The essentialist insistence that black people should identify in a particular way underpins insults such as 'bounty' or 'coconut' applied to black people (or 'banana' for Chinese-origin young people). Such names suggest that there is a core of identity beneath skin colour and that some people are not black (or 'yellow') through and through. Amina Mama (1995) discusses how such ideas caused anxiety to some of the professional black women whom she interviewed that they were not 'black enough'.

Current theorisations of identity (particularly those informed by postmodernism) construct it as plural, dynamic and situated in social contexts, rather than as static and unitary. Stuart Hall gives a clear example of how it is not possible to know how anybody will identify, simply by knowing whether they are black or white:

> In 1991, President Bush, anxious to restore a conservative majority to the US Supreme Court, nominated Clarence Thomas, a black judge of conservative political views. In Bush's judgement, white voters (who may have been prejudiced about a black judge) were likely to support Thomas because he was conservative on equal-rights legislation, and black voters (who support liberal policies on race) would support Thomas because he was black. In short, the President was 'playing the identities game'.
>
> During the Senate 'hearings' on the appointment, Judge Thomas was accused of sexual harassment by a black woman, Anita Hill, a former junior colleague of Thomas's. The hearings caused a public scandal and polarized American society. Some blacks supported Thomas on racial grounds; others opposed him on sexual grounds. Black women were divided, depending on whether their 'identities' as blacks or as women prevailed. Black men were also divided, depending on whether their sexism overrode their liberalism. White

men were divided, depending, not only on their politics, but on how they identified themselves with respect to racism and sexism. White conservative women supported Thomas, not only on political grounds, but because of their opposition to feminism. White feminists, often liberal on race, opposed Thomas on sexual grounds. And because Judge Thomas is a member of the judicial elite and Anita Hill, at the time of the alleged incident, a junior employee, there were issues of social class position at work in these arguments too.

(Hall, 1992: 279–280)

What is demonstrated in the above example is the cross-cutting and plural nature of the possible identifications that can be produced by intersections of 'race', gender and social class. Far from having static identifications and a unitary, essential identity, one person can (but does not necessarily) hold competing identifications on the basis of the different social positions they occupy. Commonalities and differences between people occupying different social positions are thus also dynamic. The appearance of black power and black consciousness movements in the 1960s (which are often cited as having had a direct impact on black children's responses in studies of 'racial identity') would seem to support theories that it is possible for there to be radical and dramatic changes in identifications and identities over the life course.

Furthermore, as discussed in the previous chapter, many people of mixed parentage are now choosing to identify themselves as definitely 'mixed' or 'biracial'. This poses challenges to the conceptualisation of black and white people as if they were binary opposites (see Root (1996) for further discussion). The 'anti-transracial adoption' position might be expected to be 'sensitive' to issues of 'race' and ethnicity, since it engages with them. However, in using static notions of racialised identities, it is insensitive to the ways in which 'race' and ethnicity are experienced and expressed. It is worth noting that, from a position in support of 'transracial adoption', Simon and her colleagues (1994) recognise that blackness is multiple and that black experience is heterogeneous. They conclude that 'transracial adoptees' are 'no less black than are children of the ghetto' (p. 115). However, the fact that they make their point of comparison 'children of the ghetto' appears to suggest that they believe that authentic blackness is really the province of the ghetto. This essentialism partly diminishes the force of their argument.

It is clear from the above discussion that theorisations of blackness used in the service of 'same-race' placement arguments are currently outdated because they are static, unitary and essentialist. In order to address the complexities now recognised to be inherent in the construction of identities, insights from psychology and other disciplines could usefully be applied. Fear that psychological arguments about identity will be used to deny racism is one reason for reluctance to use such arguments when rethinking policies and practices about children who are 'looked after' by local authorities. This is, of course, a serious issue and needs to be openly acknowledged in a context where psychological arguments are addressed, but where their potential use in the denial of racism is resisted.

Blackness is not a sufficient qualification for passing on strategies for dealing with racism

The suggestion that 'unless they are carefully trained' white adoptive parents will not be able to pass on strategies for dealing with racism to black children (Small 1986) implies that black parents, by virtue of their experiences of racism, will be able to pass on such strategies to their children. Relatively little research has been done on this issue. However, in adoption placement practice, it is not clear whether black substitute families do provide for continuity of identity for black children (Butt and Mirza, 1997).

Social work responses in the 1980s

During the 1980s the implementation of a 'same-race' placement policy involved instances of children being removed from white foster parents with whom they had spent some years. There is evidence, too, that healthy young black children spent much longer in care awaiting placement than did comparable children who were white, because of the scarcity of black adoptive parents (Chambers, 1989). However, no statistics are published, or perhaps collected, by central or local government on the ethnicity and composition of placements, or the length of time different racialised groups remain in care, or the number of placements that are disrupted by social service departments in the interests of 'racial matching'. Nor is it known to what extent practices have changed since the implementation of the 1989 Children Act. Information about such issues only becomes public in relation to individual cases, when determined foster parents have recourse to the courts, or obtain media publicity about threatened or actual removal of children. White foster parents in Liverpool, for example, who wanted to adopt a 3-year-old girl whom they had fostered for fifteen months, were told that the social work department was considering removing the child from them because she had a Jamaican great-grandfather. This somewhat bizarre proposal seems to imply an acceptance of the old US ruling that 'one drop of black blood' makes a person black. According to a spokesman for Liverpool City Council:

> Because there is a black member of the family, albeit several generations apart, our assessment of the [birth] family is that they are of mixed race. In our judgement, because of her mixed race background, her interests might be better served if she was placed with a family of similar background.

> (*Daily Telegraph*, March 17, 1990)

The positioning of social workers

The above discussion has attempted to illustrate the complexities generated by debates on 'transracial adoption' and in theories of racialised identities. These complexities are partly responsible for the difficulties social workers face in attempting to deal with the placement of children from a variety of ethnic backgrounds. The continual treatment of 'transracial adoption' as if it is a debate polarised into sides, together with the tendencies to polarise 'race' into black–white opposites, has tended to result in social workers needing to match the 'race' and/or ethnicity of parents with those of children. However, the relative poverty of social constructions of 'race' and ethnicity does not represent the plurality of backgrounds from which people come and, hence, the plurality of heritages of children to be 'looked after' by local authorities. Social workers are thus left to deal with complexities which have not been sorted out by the rest of society, and then find themselves pilloried when decisions are made which other people either do not like or consider simplistic.

This 'no-win situation' is compounded by the fact that the 'transracial adoption' debate has left social workers to surmise how to behave in a situation where rhetoric about taking 'race', racism and ethnicity seriously is not backed by commitment from managers (Rhodes, 1992). Social workers themselves have therefore not been well served by the ways in which 'transracial adoption' and fostering have been placed on the social work agenda and dealt with in practice.

Social workers are, of course, heterogeneous in their views. In a study of 835 British student social workers, for example, Kirton (1999) found that black students were markedly more likely to support 'same-race' placement than were their white colleagues. Gail Lewis (1996, 2000) and, in the Netherlands, Philomena Essed (1996), both argue that black, and minority ethnic group social workers are 'often viewed as a problem rather than an asset' (Lewis, 1996: 51). Many black social workers fear that they, together with black children and families, are in danger of being marginalised, rather than taken seriously in social work (Butt and Mirza, 1997). The fact that in 1999 social services in Brent (an area in London with a substantial black and Asian population) was found to have discriminated against black social workers whom it dismissed appears to substantiate those fears for at least some black social workers. At the same time, 'race', racism and culture are often reduced to simplistic and patronising 'culture tours' that further divide black social workers from white social workers (Lewis, 1996: 46).

> I remember when I was in Fostering and Adoption and I went on a training course 'Working with West African Families' . . . and it was a white woman running it, and 90 per cent of the people on the course were white, and they left thinking 'oh, I can work with West African families', and it was a white woman who did it. I think she had been to Nigeria twice or three times, and spent some time with a family and said 'they are so kind because they will even give you their food, even if they haven't got much, they will give it to you' in a very patronising sort of way. . . . But the thing is, ever since I have been here, I think we have had one debate on 'race' and as it so happened I was the person who had put it on the agenda.
> (African woman social worker interviewed by Gail Lewis, 1996: 46)

> The one-sided emphasis on the culture of the Other strengthens the tendency to experience ethnic groups as 'quite different' and as a 'problem'. In the meantime, people get stuck in the pattern of thinking about other cultures as a list of stereotypes: in Moroccan households, take off your shoes; don't say 'hi' to Surinamese people, but rather 'how do you do, Ma'am'; with Turks, what was it again? with Dutch people, oh great! we can be our normal selves for a change. This strengthens the familiar pattern of the Dutch being normal while others are not. You always need to show understanding for those who are not normal, whereas nobody talks about the normal.
> (Essed, 1996: 31)

In keeping with Essed's argument is the issue of whether or not social workers (mostly white, but some black) racialise 'normal' childrearing practices so that different behaviours are accepted from black than from white parents on the grounds that there are cultural differences between them (Ahmad, 1990; Lewis, 2000). This has sometimes become evident when a black child has been injured or killed by their black parents or carers. This simplistic treatment of 'race' and ethnicity as 'Other' sits side by side with attempts to privilege 'race' in childcare placements. It is perhaps not surprising that social workers find it difficult to know what is best to do in relation to 'transracial adoption' or that black social workers are often precariously positioned.

Looked-after children of mixed parentage: social policy in the twenty-first century

As the twentieth century drew to a close, governments in both Britain and the USA took steps to improve the speed and rates of adoption for all children, including those from minority ethnic groups. In the USA 'children of colour' (including black, Asian and mixed-parentage children) constitute more than 60 per cent of the children in 'out-of-home care' and wait about twice as long for adoptive homes as do other children (National Adoption Information Clearinghouse, 2001). In Britain, 89 per cent of adopters are white couples, while 20 per cent of children with an 'adoption plan' are from black or minority ethnic backgrounds. Contrary to Bebbington and Miles' (1989) estimates, it seems that although children of mixed-parentage spend longer being 'looked after' than do white children, black children who are available for adoption wait longer than those of mixed parentage. Compared with white children, children of mixed parentage wait on average eight weeks longer for placement, but black children wait on average five months longer (Department of Health, 2000; Ivaldi, 2000). This could be because local authorities are more prepared to place children of mixed parentage in white homes, but no research evidence is available on this.

It may be that children of mixed parentage spend less time in care because they are more likely to have 'lighter skin'. McRoy and Grape (1999) found that skin colour is still an important factor in the USA for parents' choice of an adoptive child and that this was true for black as well as white adoptive parents. This echoes a finding discussed by Tizard (1991) in her review of intercountry adoptions – that adopters tended to prefer children who were as near white as possible. It also complements the accounts of some black women in Mama's (1995) study, who felt that, in their childhoods, they had been made to feel that their skin colour was too dark to be acceptable or attractive. However, Hollingsworth (1998) argues that the more similar an adopted child to their adopted family, the more satisfactory is the adoption and the adjustment of the adopted child.

Two studies which involved the examination of the case files of over a hundred children of mixed parentage before they came into care found that most had lived with lone white mothers who were in receipt of state benefit in local authority housing (Barn, 1993, 1999; Barn *et al.*, 1997). Barn argues that the Asian and African Caribbean children whose files they examined were always matched for ethnicity to the families in which they were placed, but that few of the 'mixed-race' children were placed in mixed families. They were as likely to be placed in white families as in black families. This caused dilemmas for social workers who sometimes engaged in discussions around the children's shades of colour. The question of who it is appropriate for children of mixed parentage to be placed with is one that the study which informs this book can throw some light on.

In the USA, various court judgments in favour of white parents wanting to adopt African American children together with the advocacy of some researchers of 'transracial adoption' (e.g. Bagley, 1993; Silverman, 1993; Simon and Alstein, 1996) and concern about the numbers of African American children in foster care led to the Multi-Ethnic Placement Act (1994) and the Interethnic Adoption Provisions (1996). These both aimed to remove 'race-related' considerations, with the 1996 provisions instructing that 'race' cannot be routinely used when making placement decisions. In Texas, USA, 'state law stipulates that any employee who attempts to remove a child from transracial family foster care for the purpose of same-race adoptive placement or who denies or delays a placement in order to seek a same-race family is subject to immediate dismissal' (McRoy and Grape, 1999: 674).

In Britain, the 'New Labour' government elected in 1997 also aimed to reduce the number of children being 'looked after' long term in local authority care. However, in much the same way that the Children Act 1989 did, the Adoption Bill which they introduced in 2001 leaves more space for interpretation than does the USA legislation.

Children's birth heritage and religious, cultural and linguistic background are all important factors to consider in finding them a new family. The Department of Health circular LAC (98) 20 states that the best family for a child will be one that best reflects their birth heritage, and all councils should be proactive in monitoring their local population of looked after children to enable them to recruit permanent carers who can meet their needs. However, the child's welfare is paramount, and no child should be denied loving adoptive parents solely on the grounds that the child and the parents do not share the same racial or cultural background.

(Section 6.15 in *Adoption: A New Approach*. White Paper, December 2000)

This of course leaves open what should be counted as appropriate heritage (and so 'same-race' placement) for children of mixed parentage, as well as how much attention to give to issues of racism and culture in 'transracial placements'. However, it accords with the growing number of researchers who argue that the ideal practice is 'same-race' placement, but that the best available solution is 'transracial adoption' if children would otherwise have to wait for long periods for adoptive homes (e.g. Haugaard, 2000).

It is due to the strong feeling against 'transracial adoption' for over two decades that there has been a reduction in the numbers of 'transracial adoptions' in Britain. Figures published by the British Agencies on Adoption and Fostering indicate that in 1995, 24 per cent of the adoptions recorded by local authorities and 6 per cent of those reported by voluntary agencies were 'transracial' placements (BAAF, 1997). Although national figures are not available, this compares with 71 per cent of black and mixed-parentage children who were placed with two white parents in a study done in the early 1980s (Thoburn *et al.*, 2000).

However, what is meant by 'same-race' placement and what is considered to be the achievement of 'matching' has often been muddy. For example, Thoburn and Moffatt (2001) found that children of two directly African parents had been placed with black parents, but never with two African parents. There seemed to be a 'belief that colour was a more significant consideration than race, ethnicity or culture, except possibly with respect to religion' (Department of Health, 1999: 43). There are, of course, good reasons for privileging racialisation over ethnicisation in placement decisions since, if concerns about dealing with racism are foremost, black parents are likely to have experienced racism in similar ways to black children. However, this raises the issue of whether or not black parents generally pass on ideas about how to cope with racism to their children. Moreover, there are often ideas about cultural transmission that are meaningless if adoptive parents and children come from different ethnic groups that treat culture in unitary, static ways. The difficulties faced by agencies placing children for adoption alert us to the possibility that while 'transracial' placements have reduced in Britain, the issue of 'matching' is not necessarily settled.

Importantly for a consideration of mixed parentage, Quinton *et al.*

(1998) found that one in six of the children in their study were from minority ethnic backgrounds and half of them had been 'ethnically matched'. However, all except one of those who had not been 'ethnically matched' were of mixed parentage, with many having been brought up by white mothers in predominantly white contexts. This raises the question of what is being considered as ethnic matching and whether or not it is relevant given that children of mixed parentage who are not 'looked after' by local authorities live in a variety of households in relation to ethnicity. Thoburn *et al.* (2000) asked adults who had been 'transracially adopted' (whom they had first studied almost two decades before) how they felt about 'same-race' or 'transracial' placements. Children of mixed parentage appeared to feel less strongly about this than did black children.

The way forward?

While the 'transracial adoption' debate is often presented in its strong form, as polarised sides, many people who locate themselves on one or other side recognise that, since social circumstances are never perfect, it may be necessary to make placements with which, in ideal circumstances, they would disagree. In addition, those who are politically 'worlds apart' may sometimes share the same positions with regard to 'transracial adoption'. Nonetheless, one important benefit provided by the raising of the 'transracial adoption' debate, has been the placing of 'race', ethnicity and racism on the social work agenda. As a result, a 'colour-blind' approach is less tenable now than in the past.

The intricacy of the issues raised by 'transracial adoption' makes it unlikely that easy ways may be found to implement insights from psychology (and other disciplines) in practice. It is clear from psychological work that racialised identities are more complex than opponents of 'transracial adoption' have tended to allow. In being apparently 'sensitive' to 'race' and ethnicity, they have been insensitive to the ways in which 'race' and ethnicity are represented in identities. Supporters of 'transracial adoption' are, however, unjustified in using criticisms of the 'anti-transracial adoption' position as justification for a 'colour- (and ethnicity-)blind' approach. Other psychological work indicates that 'race', ethnicity and racism are important from early on in children's lives (e.g. Bath and Farrell, 1996). Furthermore, the ways in which racism impacts on black social workers can easily serve to marginalise their (plural) viewpoints (Lewis, 2000). Failure to recognise this would further justify a retreat from addressing issues of 'race' and racism (Kirton, 1996), allowing psychological evidence to be used for the maintenance of the political status quo. 'Transracial adoption' provides perhaps the most vivid example of how politics and psychology intersect in social work theory and practice. It is this that makes the controversy a recursive one.

Recent research on social care in Britain indicates that while controversies abound in all aspects of the care of black children and their families' experiences, it is possible to produce clear and practical suggestions for improvements in practice (Barn, 1993; Butt and Mirza, 1997; Jones and Butt, 1995). Almost all the US publications on 'transracial adoption' similarly make policy recommendations. In order for this to happen, any theoretically informed social work practice has to engage both with the impact of racism and with the dynamic pluralism of racialised identities. Both have to be taken on board in decisions about the placement of children. But decisions cannot simply be 'colour coded'. Using psychological evidence in order to be genuinely sensitive to 'race' and ethnicity requires an engagement with the complexities of 'transracial adoption'.

It is clear that the 'transracial adoption' debate is far from closed. As we have seen, some researchers now question the methodological soundness of many studies that provided support for 'transracial adoption' (Alexander and Curtis, 1996; Hollingsworth, 1997; Park and Green, 2000). Many researchers agree that more research is needed to inform practice which recognises that 'race' is socially important and takes account of the specific needs of children – including those of mixed parentage (e.g. Banks, 1995; McRoy, 1994).

Framework for a study of mixed-parentage adolescents

Given the continuing lack of clarity about 'transracial adoption', and the disagreement about how mixed-parentage children should be placed, we believe that the study reported in this book makes a contribution to understanding the background issues to debates about 'transracial adoption'. There has been very little research on the identity of mixed-parentage adolescents living with their own parents, and none on their cultural ties, or ability to cope with racism. We decided, therefore, that as the next step in the debate it was important to remedy these omissions, especially since we knew that many mixed-parentage children living with their white birth mother, and sometimes white stepfather, are being brought up, like 'transracially adopted' children, without a black parent.

Moreover, quite apart from the implications for 'transracial adoption' of studying non-adopted mixed-parentage adolescents, it seemed important to explore their racialised identities in a society which, while still in many ways racist, has markedly changed in the past thirty years. The biggest changes have probably occurred in local authority secondary schools in cities. Before it was abolished, the Inner London Education Authority, in particular, formulated a strong antiracist policy in the early 1980s. It required each school to make a 'clear, unambiguous statement of opposition to any form of racism or racist behaviour, and . . . [to provide] an explanation of the way in which the school or college intends to develop practices which tackle racism' (ILEA, 1983).

While there is often a gap between policy and practice and there is still a great deal of racialised informal segregation in schools (e.g. Frosh *et al.*, 2001; Phoenix, 1998), it is important to explore the changes that have occurred. As well as changes in educational policy, there is evidence from anthropological and sociological work (Back, 1996; Hewitt, 1986; Jones, 1988) that the newly developed black youth cultures are much admired by sectors of white youth. It seemed possible that these changes have produced a social environment within some London secondary schools where young people of mixed parentage might feel positive about their origins. If this is so, it strengthens the case of those who argue that white families who adopt black and mixed-parentage children should live in ethnically mixed neighbourhoods and send them to ethnically mixed schools (e.g. McRoy and Zurcher, 1983).

From the point of view of both policy and theory, we also thought it important to explore a hitherto neglected issue; that is, the extent to which adolescents' racialised and cultural identities are influenced by their gender and social class. In the past, as we showed in Chapter 2, attitudes to black people have at certain times and in certain social contexts been strongly influenced by both these factors and, if this is the case today, it is likely to be reflected in their identities. Gender and social class also influence the cultural allegiances of young people; to the extent that black youth cultures can be identified, we would expect allegiance to it to be related to gender and social class as well as 'race'. In relation to transracial origin, not only were the young people whom we interviewed not being 'looked after' by local authorities, they were also not predominantly living in poverty (unlike many children at the point at which a local authority takes responsibility for their care). While this may be seen as a shortcoming for answering questions about 'transracial adoption', it does help to sort out which issues are particularly to do with identity and mixed parentage and which are related to sociostructural positioning.

Since parental teaching and influence have been considered a crucial influence on racialised identity in the 'transracial adoption' debate and on 'coping skills', we also thought it important to interview some of the young people's parents. We explored with them the ways in which they have attempted to influence their children's racialised identity, and to find out what 'coping strategies' they have passed on to them, whether implicitly or explicitly. The findings in the chapters that follow also throw light on how children's allegiances to their parents and social experiences would affect their choice of which racialised 'side' to take if they had to make a forced choice. They give some indication of differences in the racialised allegiances of children of mixed parentage. Recognition of such differences serves to remind us that the complexity of the transracial debate for children of mixed parentage partly results from the everyday racialised complexities they face. Overall, then, the findings from this study provide background information that can be used to inform the 'transracial adoption' debate.

5 How the research was carried out

In this chapter we describe how we chose the young people for the study, what kinds of schools and families they came from, and how we interviewed them and analysed our findings. The interviews were carried out in 1990–91, shortly before the first edition of this book was published. The findings are described in Chapter 6 onwards.

Selection of young people

Our research into the racialised identities of young people of mixed parentage, living with their birth parents, was part of a wider study which included two other groups of young people: those with two white British parents, and those with two black parents of African Caribbean origin. This wider study included fieldwork carried out in two London youth clubs by Les Back (1991a, 1991b) as well as an interview study. In this book we focus on the mixed-parentage group, although in this chapter we describe the methodology of the whole interview study.

Because we wanted to study as representative a sample as possible, we decided to locate our sample through the school system, and to interview young people aged 15–16 in the fifth year of secondary school. If we had selected the sixth year, we would have missed the less academic students, since at least half the students would have left school at 16, and thereafter would have been very difficult to locate. Below the fifth year, we thought that the young people might not be sufficiently self-aware and articulate to deal with questions about their identity, and would be less likely to be concerned with such issues as employment prospects and their own future.

Since we expected that both gender and social class would be important influences on identity, we needed to interview both boys and girls, and those from middle-class families as well as those from working-class families. We decided to confine our research to black, white and mixed-parentage young people, because we were interested in the possible implications of the findings for the issue of transracial adoption and fostering. Mixed-parentage children in particular are the group most likely to be found in long-term care, and to be placed for adoption (Rowe *et al.*, 1989). Unfortunately, we did not have sufficient resources to add on other groups, such as young people of Asian origin, despite our interest in them. We planned, therefore, that our sample would be made up of sixty young white people, sixty black (with two African Caribbean parents) and sixty of mixed-parentage, that is, with one white and one black African or African Caribbean parent. Each group would include equal numbers of boys and girls from working-class and middle-class families aged 15–16. Since we intended to interview the young people individually for at least an hour, our resources would not stretch to a larger sample. But we decided it was more important to encourage the young people to talk freely and at length than to carry out a brief survey with larger numbers. We also hoped to interview the parents of about half of them.

Where we found the young people

Having decided on the kind of young people we wanted to interview, our next step was to find them. We decided to select children from a number of schools, rather than from just a few. This was because we wanted to include different types of school in the study, both multi-racial and predominantly white schools, and single-sex as well as coeducational schools. In each school, we hoped to interview black, white and mixed-parentage fifth-formers, from both working-class and middle-class homes.

After obtaining permission from five education authorities in central and outer London, we approached the heads of their secondary schools for permission to interview their students. While we received few outright refusals, there is no doubt that many heads were wary of research on racialised issues. The conditions imposed by some heads, and the delays in granting permission that occurred in other schools, meant that we only worked in about one-third of the schools we approached.

It was soon clear that our original neat plan was unrealistic. A few schools, while otherwise welcoming, would not allow us to interview fifth-formers, since this was the examination year for GCSE; in these instances we interviewed young people in their final term of the fourth year or their first term of the sixth year. Some schools had no students of the right age from middle-class families, and boys' schools were more often unwilling to allow us to interview their students than girls' schools. It was particularly difficult to find young black people from middle-class families. Unlike the situation in the USA, analysis of recent Labour Force Survey data has shown that the black middle class in Britain is still very small, although growing (Charlie Owen, personal communication). Mixed-parentage young people of any social class were also hard to find. This is because, as we described in Chapter 2, although their numbers are rapidly growing, *more than half* of all the mixed-parentage people in Britain are under the age of 10.

Because of the difficulty in locating middle-class black and mixed-parentage young people, we decided to ask all the larger independent (private) schools in London and the Home Counties whether they had any black or mixed-parentage students of the right age, and, if so, whether we could interview them, together with one or more white students of the same sex, and nearest in age. Many of the schools did not have such students, and others, mainly boys' schools, were not willing to give us access; of the independent schools which took part in the study, only one-fifth were boys' schools. In the end we almost reached our target number of sixty mixed-parentage young people, and well exceeded it in the case of the young black and white people. However, we had more girls than boys, especially in the white and mixed-parentage groups.

Contacting the parents was not a simple matter, since most head-teachers were unwilling to act as intermediaries. We decided to ask the young people at the end of the interview whether they would mind if we interviewed their parents, and if not, whether they would give us their address and phone number. A substantial number said that they *did* mind, or that their parents were too busy, etc. It seems likely that, despite our assurances of confidentiality, they were worried that some of their comments might be repeated. Of those parents whom we were able to approach, very few declined to be interviewed, but a number had to be abandoned because they kept postponing appointments. In the end, we were able to interview only one-third of the parents, rather than the half we had originally intended, and they were clearly a self-selected sample.

The mixed-parentage sample

The mixed-parentage sample was made up of fifty-eight young people attending thirty-two different schools. Nearly three-quarters (72 per cent) were girls, and 73 per cent were aged 15 or 16, with approximately equal numbers of the rest being older or younger. Table 5.1 (see Appendix) shows that half – 55 per cent – attended independent schools where in all but one case the students were predominantly white. The local authority schools attended by the rest were almost all racially mixed. A 'predominantly white' school was one where we estimated that about 75 per cent or more of the students in the fifth year were white. (The schools did not keep ethnic statistics, and the proportion of white students varied, sometimes markedly, from one year to another, so the classification of the schools is only approximate.) In the predominantly white schools there were usually only one or two students of African or African Caribbean origin in the year, sometimes in the whole school, although there was often a substantial minority of students of Asian and Middle Eastern origin. The racially mixed comprehensive schools varied widely in their composition, some having a majority of pupils of Asian origin, others of African Caribbean origin, while in others the proportions of white, black and Asian students were about equal. Two-thirds of the young people were attending either single-sex schools, or schools where there was a preponderance of boys.

Table 5.2 (see Appendix) shows that 61 per cent of the fathers (or, in single parent families, the mothers) were in professional or managerial occupations (social class 1 or 2). While three-quarters of the mothers were white, the majority of the fathers (69 per cent) were black, usually from the Caribbean. Only two black parents had been born in the UK, compared with 88 per cent of their children.

Table 5.3 (see Appendix) shows that 57 per cent of the young people lived with both their parents; the next most common arrangement was to live with a single mother. Sixty per cent of the sample lived with a white and a black parent or step-parent, 28 per cent with a single white parent or step-parent, and 12 per cent with a black parent or black parent and step-parent only (Table 5.4: see Appendix). We wanted to compare those who lived with a white parent or parents only with those who lived with a black parent. Because the proportion of those living with a black parent only was so small, for the purpose of our analysis we grouped them with those who were living with one black and one white parent. We contrasted them with the rest of the sample (28 per cent) who lived with no black parents, i.e. with a white single parent or a white parent and white step-parent.

The interviews

The interviews were designed by the authors, one of whom is black, the other white, and piloted extensively before the main study began. They were composed mainly of open-ended questions which allow the respondent to answer freely, rather than having to select one of several specified alternatives, as in a survey. The wording of the questions, and the order in which they were asked, were determined in advance, although the interviewer was free to add supplementary questions if the answers were not clear. There were sections on gender and social class identity before the section on racialised identity and racism, which was the longest, and which was followed by questions on friendship, religion and national identity. Half of the interviews lasted between an hour and an hour and a half, with about a quarter lasting less than this, and a quarter more. Almost all the interviews with the young people took place in their schools, usually in an empty classroom. The interviews with the parents are described in Chapter 9.

At the end of the interview we asked the young people how they felt about it, and whether there were any questions *they* would like to ask. Half of the mixed-parentage young people were definitely positive about the interview (e.g. 'I enjoyed it very much'; 'I thought it was interesting, 'cos I've never actually thought about some of the questions before'); a quarter made neutral comments (e.g. 'It was all right'; 'I didn't mind it'); one-fifth had mixed feelings (e.g. 'I felt nervous, it got a bit easier as it went on, I didn't mind it'); while two young people said they hadn't enjoyed it. Just over half accepted the invitation to ask questions themselves, generally 'What is all this for? What will you do with the results?' Some young people from all three racialised groups turned the tables on the black interviewers, and asked them about *their* experiences of racism, relationships with white people, whether they had experienced problems in getting a job, etc. They seemed genuinely curious, and in some cases, perhaps, were seeking reassurance.

The interviews with the parents took place in their homes. They included many of the questions we had asked their children, but also questions on whether and how they had attempted to influence their children's views and their strategies for helping their children to cope with racism. Most parents had a great deal to say, and the interviews generally lasted between two and three hours. We asked, and received, permission both from the parents and their children to tape-record the interviews.

Many of our findings come from straightforward quantitative analyses; for example, counting the number of young people who said they would prefer to be another colour, or who said they had been subjected to racist abuse. For other analyses, especially those relating to racialised identity and ways of dealing with racism, we needed the transcripts of the tape-recordings in order to use the detailed accounts the young people gave of their experiences, both in their answers and in their spontaneous comments throughout the interview.

There is evidence, mainly from the USA, that both black and white people tend to give different answers to questions with a racial content according to the race of the interviewer (Schaeffer, 1980). Previous British research with mixed-parentage children has been criticised for using white interviewers, so since no mixed-race interviewers were available we endeavoured to use black interviewers. For logistical reasons this was not always possible, but the great majority – 78 per cent – of the interviews with the young people of mixed parentage were carried out by two black women, the rest by two white women. In the case of the parents, 61 per cent of the interviews, including all those with black parents, were carried out by the two black interviewers.

Strengths and limitations of the sample

A major difficulty in studying people of mixed parentage is in locating a representative sample. Previous researchers have generally found mixed-parentage people through social networks, starting with inter-racial organisations, such as 'Harmony', or in some cases through advertising, but these procedures are likely to produce a sample with a particular point of view. The strength of our sample is that it was located through the school system and was not made up of volunteers, but of those young people who were selected by the staff as fitting our categories and who were present when we visited the schools. Working in thirty-four schools of different types ensured that our findings would not be biased by the characteristics of individual schools, and allowed us to compare the accounts of students attending state and independent schools, and schools of different racial composition.

Sixty-one per cent of our sample came from middle-class families, and half attended independent schools. Since only 8.5 per cent of secondary school-aged pupils attend independent schools (Department of Education and Science, 1991) and only 31 per cent of men, and many fewer black men, are in social class 1 and 2 (OPCS, 1992), our sample is clearly overweighted with middle-class families, compared with the national average. However, since the social class distribution of mixed black and white couples in the country as a whole is not known, we do not know the extent to which our sample is unrepresentative of them. Although it tends to be assumed that mixed-parentage children come from working-class families, this may not be the case. In the USA they are usually born into professional, middle-class families (Spickard, 1989: 293). There is no evidence available, either, with which we could judge whether the proportion of young people in single-parent families in our sample (one-third) is representative of mixed-parentage young people in general in England.

The objection may be made that because 60 per cent of the sample is middle class, the findings are not relevant to social workers. However, as we will describe below, our sample enabled us to show the ways in which the experience of being of mixed parentage is mediated by social class. This analysis is very relevant to social workers. For example, foster and adoptive homes are often middle class, and social workers may worry that transracially placed children are not as 'black' as their non-adopted counterparts, when they are, in fact, compared to black working-class, rather than middle-class, children. In a number of important respects, however, we found no social class differences among the mixed-parentage sample, and these findings are directly relevant to social work practice.

A real problem with our sample is the serious under-representation of boys, which seems to have resulted from the reluctance of boys' schools, especially boys' independent schools, to take part in the study. Because boys more often reported experiencing racism than girls, the gender imbalance is likely to have led to an under-representation of the amount of racism suffered by mixed-parentage young people (Chapter 7). It might also be claimed that our sample size of fifty-eight mixed-parentage young people is very small, but if it had been much larger we would not have been able to analyse in such detail the verbatim accounts which the young people gave of their feelings and experiences. Another possible limitation to generalisability is the London base of the sample, but this can also be seen as an advantage. London is a multiracial city, with the largest concentration of people of Caribbean origin in Britain, where both the Greater London council and the Inner London Education Authority pursued an anti-racist policy, prior to being abolished. By confining our study to the London region we were able to see the impact on the young people's identity of these relatively favourable influences.

6 The racialised identities of the young people of mixed parentage

In Chapter 2 we pointed out that there has been virtually no research about the racialised identity of adolescents of mixed parentage living in their own families. We decided to explore four aspects of this topic with the young people in our study:

1 whether they regarded themselves as black;
2 whether they felt positive or negative or confused about their mixed parentage;
3 the extent to which their racialised identity was central in their lives;
4 the extent to which they felt an affinity to black cultures, and to black and white people.

We explored these issues at various times during the interview, in order to allow the young people to have second thoughts or to enlarge on an earlier response. In this chapter we will discuss their answers in relation to the first three issues.

Did the young people regard themselves as black?

As we saw in Chapter 2, much recent discussion about the identity of mixed-parentage children has centred around the issue of whether they 'correctly' label themselves. Increasingly, it has been argued by many social workers and some black people that their identity 'should' be black, since they are regarded as black by white people. If they fail to regard themselves as black, they are said to be denying reality, with all the risks that denial carries of psychological damage. Mixed-parentage children growing up in white families are thought to be in particular danger of thinking of themselves as white.

We explored the issue of how the young people defined themselves by asking the following questions: 'Do you ever use the term "black" for people? Who do you include in this term? Do you include people with one white and one black parent? Do you ever use the term "coloured"? Who do you include as coloured?' And, if not already apparent, 'What do you call people with one black parent and one white parent?' Later in the interview we asked, 'You said that you call people with one black and one white parent – but do you think of yourself as black?' We were careful to note early on in the interview which 'racial' terms they used themselves, either spontaneously or in response to a question, and thereafter to use their terms in talking to them.

All but two of the young people (who preferred the term 'coloured') said they did use the term 'black'. However, just over half (54 per cent) did not use the term for people of mixed parentage: they confined its use to people with two African or African Caribbean parents (Table 6.1: see Appendix). The rest (46 per cent) did include mixed-parentage people with Africans and African Caribbeans as 'black'. Only 12 per cent used the term 'black' to include Asians, and only one person gave 'black' the more general meaning of 'anybody not white'.

Later in the interview we rephrased the question, and asked the young people whether they regarded *themselves* as black. Several who had said earlier in the interview that they called people with one white and one black parent 'black', at this point said they did not think of themselves as black. One girl, for example, who had answered 'I suppose so, yes' to the earlier question, replied to the later question, 'No, not really, but I don't think of myself as white, either'. Another, who had answered 'Yes, society treats me as black' to the first question, answered to the second: 'No, I don't think of myself as black, exactly, I think of myself as half-British, half-Jamaican, though essentially I feel myself to be British, because I was born here.' Overall, 39 per cent said they thought of themselves as black, a further 10 per cent saying they did so in certain situations, while 49 per cent said they did not.

Many of the young people seemed to have given a lot of thought to the issue. Some of those who did not call themselves black said that to do so would be to deny their white ancestry. One girl, living with a single white mother, said:

'I wouldn't call myself black. I mean, lots of people have said if you are mixed race you might just as well call yourself black, but I feel that is denying the fact that my mother is white, and I'm not going to do that.'

Another girl, living with a single black mother, said she did call herself black, but was rethinking the issue. The following quotation exemplifies the process of identity change, in this case a transition from a black to a mixed identity:

> 'No. Yes. Yeah, mainly because I'm conditioned to do that [call self black]. I mean, I'm half, and most of my friends have been white, so they call me black, but nowadays I'm thinking more towards, well I'm half black, but then I'm half white.'

Most of the young people who called themselves black did not elaborate on why they did so. However, it was clear that some were aware of current thinking on the issue. One girl, who lived with both of her parents, said:

> 'At first I only included African Caribbeans or Africans, but now I realise [black] is a word that's much more ambiguous than your colour or your features or anything, it includes an attitude of white people towards black people and black people towards themselves. . . . As far as the white person is concerned black is "other", they'll see someone other than white coming down the street, so that's what made me realise I'm black.'

Those who did not call themselves black usually called themselves 'brown', 'half-and-half', 'mixed' or 'coloured'. The term 'coloured', elsewhere formerly used to refer to anyone who was not white, was slated by the black consciousness movement in the 1960s and 1970s, and the term 'black' was substituted. This substitution took place not, as some of our young people believed, because 'coloured' was an absurd descriptive term, but as part of a political struggle. The category 'black' was intended to unite all racially oppressed peoples, and to affirm pride in a stigmatised group. However, we found that 'coloured' was still widely used. Forty-three per cent of the mixed-parentage sample used it, as did 30 per cent of the black sample, and 61 per cent of the white (Table 6.1). It was mainly used as a term for anyone who was not white, but a minority confined it to people of mixed parentage and Asian people.

The 57 per cent who did not use the term 'coloured' tended to react quite strongly against it. One girl who lived with a single white mother, said:

> 'I really hate the word, it's really stupid, I mean, when you think about it really logically, coloured could be any colour, blue, yellow,

green, red. I mean people just aren't that colour, I think it's ridiculous.'

Others made the point that 'white people are coloured too, they're just not darkly coloured'. Those who did use the term tended to see it as a less 'harsh' term than black. Thus one boy who lived with a white mother, said:

'I just think it sounds less harsh, somehow. It's, I don't know really, it doesn't sound offensive for some reason. I know that a lot of African Caribbeans and Africans prefer to be called black than coloured, I don't know why, but, you know, that's what I've heard.'

Others had acquired the term from an older Caribbean-born generation, to whom the term 'black' was still offensive. One girl, although she did not use the term herself, was sympathetic to those who did.

'I don't think it's a wrong word [coloured]. People don't like the word "black", they're frightened of it, I think. And I remember that my West Indian granny told me not to use the word "black", she said "brown" or "coloured", not black.'

Some young people adapted their terminology to whatever they felt was appropriate to the situation. Asked whether he used the term 'coloured', a boy who lived with his black father and white mother said:

'Well, at home, really. Sometimes I use the word "black" at school, it don't seem to be offensive. I think my dad's a bit funny on the term "black". He don't say nothing, but every time I say it he looks at me or something like that in a serious way. So I just stopped saying it at home. [*But you say it outside, at school?*] Yes, most of the time, 'cos other people outside use it, so I just use it.'

A smaller number of young people described themselves as 'brown', either instead of, or as well as, 'coloured'. And a small proportion – 16 per cent – seemed very uncertain in their use of colour names; all those in this group lived with a black parent.

None of the young people described themselves as white, but 10 per cent (six) said they felt 'more white than black' or that they sometimes thought of themselves as white. All six were living with a black parent. Three were considered by the interviewers to look white. They did not call themselves or other people of mixed parentage black, preferring to explain that they had one white and one black parent. One boy said he thought of himself as white because no one would think he was black if they had not known he had a black father. When asked if there were any circumstances in which he thought of himself as black he made a distinction between his identity, which was not black, and his black ancestry (blood).

> 'Not as being black, but of having black blood. If I'm in a family group of my dad's family, I suppose then I might feel black, but otherwise I don't really think so.'

Another girl who looked white made the point that her identity differed in different situations:

> 'Sometimes I think of myself as being English, and sometimes I think of myself as being more Afr . . . well, kind of African, it depends on the situation a lot. And sometimes I think of myself as being neither, really just being like tanned, a tanned British person.'

The other three who said they sometimes thought of themselves as white did not look white, but they got on badly with their black parent, and had a very strong relationship with their white parent. One of these young people had constructed an identity for himself as a 'dark' white person, which involved a belief that white people differ from black in personality and views, as well as colour.

> 'Half the time, I sort of feel myself as a white person, but with a darker skin, and I sort of forget exactly what colour I am. When I say "white", I mean the personality, because you'll find like black people have different views on things.'

Another said:

> 'When I hear people saying nasty things about black people then I'll sit there and I'll think, well I'm half black, you know, and sometimes I just don't feel as if I'm black, and I'll start to think about it, I don't know, I see myself as more white than black, especially in certain situations, I do.'

Half of the young people, then, described themselves as having an intermediate identity, neither black nor white. We tried to see whether, in a hypothetical situation in which black and white people were described as being in conflict, more of the young people would identify with one group or another. However, their answers only marginally altered their previous identification. Forty-one per cent said they would side with the black people, 38 per cent refused to make a choice, saying that it would depend on the issue, or that they could not choose, while 13 per cent said they would side with the white people. One girl said:

> 'Do I have to choose? I'll say black. Because I think black people definitely have been more oppressed than white people, and they may need more encouragement and I also feel that because I am brown I can help because I know a bit of what the other side thinks like.'

Many of the young people interpreted the hypothetical conflict in terms of their own family relationships:

> 'If it meant having to take a side, I think I would end up taking the white side, because the white side is the family I love. I do love my black family, but I love my white family more.'

> 'Well, I'd be alienating one of my parents if I chose, and I wouldn't want to do that. I think I'd be on the side that accepted me, rather than choosing sides.'

> 'I think I'd most probably go on the black side. But if it has to happen to my Mum and Dad as well, no, I think I'd go with my Mum on the white side.'

Mixed race, mixed parentage, or half-caste?

The great majority (79 per cent) of the young people, as well as calling themselves black, brown or coloured, used another term which referred to their mixed ancestry. We noted in Chapter 4 that from the 1960s and 1970s onwards some black people objected to the use of the term 'half-caste'. They argued that such people should generally simply be referred to as black, but if an additional label was necessary for a specific purpose, 'mixed race' should be used. Subsequently it was argued that 'mixed parentage' was a preferable term.

However, we found that these newer terms had not yet been generally adopted in London secondary schools. Forty-three per cent of the mixed-parentage young people used the term 'half-caste', as did 57 per cent of the black sample and 61 per cent of the white. Only 24 per cent of the mixed-parentage young people used the term 'mixed race', and a further 12 per cent said they used both terms (Table 6.1). None used the term 'mixed parentage'. We were surprised to find that the term 'negro', which we had thought was obsolete, was used by five young people of mixed parentage to refer to people with two black parents. (These five young people all lived with a black parent, and attended independent schools.)

A number of the young people were aware that some adults disliked the term 'half-caste', but they preferred to stick with the term in use in their social circle. One girl who lived with both her parents resisted considerable adult pressure on her to alter her terminology.

> 'I call myself half-caste, but my Mum doesn't like it, my teachers don't like it. [*Why?*] My Mum thinks it's a horrible word, the teacher at school, he's black, he just says it's a horrible thing to say about yourself, it's like implying you're a dog. He says; "No, you're black". [*And your dad?*] He says I'm black, too.'

Often the young people did not know, or had misunderstood, the objections to the term. One boy, after describing himself as half-caste, said:

> 'I think it should be mixed race or something, but I've been brought up with the word half-caste. [*Why should it be mixed race?*] 'Cos this woman said it's actually called mixed race, half-caste is sort of like the wrong word, as if you've been casted, like.'

Others adapted their terminology to the situation. A number of the young people seemed to view the term 'half-caste' as informal, and suitable for use with peers, while 'mixed race' was kept for formal use. Thus, one girl who lived with both her parents commented:

> 'I just say half-caste if I'm around, you know, my friends, but if I'm talking to someone like yourself I say mixed race.'

Similarly, a boy who lived with his single white mother commented:

> 'If I was writing a job application or something I'd put mixed race, but I think half-caste is more sort of, more of a relaxed term, you know.'

Those who preferred the term 'mixed race' gave a variety of reasons for preferring it. One girl who lived with her white mother said:

'My mum always said that half-caste didn't sound nice, and when I think about it, it makes you feel like you are half-and-half, and I think mixed race sounds nice because it sounds as if you are mixed, which I am, but not as if you are half a person.'

Another girl who lived with her black mother, said:

'I won't use the term "half-caste" again because my mum has pointed out to me that it's a racist word. I don't mind people using it, I don't get angry if people use this word, because half-caste is a very widely used word, and people don't actually realise what it means, it means half-made, actually, half white and half another, worse, culture, or whatever, and I don't use that word.'

A third girl said:

'I used to say half-caste, but someone told me that was wrong, because caste apparently means class, so it sounds like, you know, black people are in the lower class, perhaps.'

About one-fifth (twelve) of the young people of mixed parentage did not use either term. Most of these simply called people of mixed parentage 'coloured' or 'brown' or 'black', while the rest had no general term, but described people according to their specific origins. Thus one girl said:

'I just say that they've got a British mother and an African father, or whatever, I don't use a special word.'

Black or half-caste: what factors influenced the choice of labels?

For the whole sample, including the black and white groups, the use of the term 'half-caste' was strongly associated with social class. Young people from a working-class background were much more likely to use the term 'half-caste' than 'mixed race' (71 per cent did so, against 43 per cent of middle-class young people). Those from a middle-class background were more likely to use the term 'mixed race'.

Social class did not, however, influence their use of the term 'coloured', or whether they called people of mixed parentage 'black', nor did the 'racial' composition of the family or the school. Young people of mixed parentage who lived with a single white parent, or white parent and step-parent, did not differ in their use of any 'racial' terms from those who lived with a single black parent or black parent and step-parent, or from those who lived with both parents. These findings do not mean that their parents did not influence the young people's racialised identity, but the direction of the influence was not related to their colour or social class. Sometimes the two parents attempted to influence them in opposite directions.

> 'My mum [white] has always brought me up to say, if anyone asks you what colour you are, you tell them you're black, because no matter what, if you walk down the street someone will look at you and say, "Oh, there's a black girl". My dad [black] has always said to me, "You're not black and you're not white, say what you are if anyone asks you, you are mixed race, you've got nothing to be ashamed of". But then my mum says, "No, you are black".'

Defining themselves as 'black' was strongly related to a set of attitudes about racism which were more politicised than those of the young people who did not use the term (Table 6.2: see Appendix). Specifically, those young people of mixed parentage who said they thought of themselves as black tended not to use the terms 'coloured' and 'half-caste'. They tended to describe racism as coming only from white people, rather than saying 'anyone can be racist'; to say that name-calling is always racist, rather than that it depends on the circumstances; and to believe that if they had been white both their past and their future lives would be easier, and, had they been black, more difficult.

Holding these views was not related to living with a black parent – they were often held by young people living in an otherwise all-white household. They *were* related to attending a state rather than independent school, and with describing more experience of racism (Table 6.3: see Appendix).

There was some evidence that the young people's appearance also influenced their identity, since of the nine young people who looked white only one said they thought of themselves as black. We suspected, also, that there was a tendency for those who had a good relationship with one parent and a very poor relationship with the other to identify 'racially' with the former. However, since the interview was not designed to study parent–child relationships, we do not have systematic evidence on this point.

Did the young people feel positive about their mixed parentage?

According to some theorising (popularised within social work from the 1970s onwards), a positive image for mixed-parentage people can come only from assuming a black identity, and identifying with other black people. By implication, this involves rejecting their white inheritance. Marginality theory, also, would predict that those who identified with neither black nor white groups would have a negative identity, feeling rejected by both. Since under half of our sample regarded themselves as black we were able to explore these theories in a series of questions asked quite late in the interview. By this time they had discussed their experience of racism (see Chapter 8), so that any unhappy feelings about their colour were likely to have surfaced, and might be more easily expressed than if we had asked the questions 'from cold'.

The past

First we asked them whether they had ever in the past – perhaps when they were very young – wished they were another colour. Half (51 per cent) said they had (Table 6.4: see Appendix). Of these, thirteen young people said they had often wished it, and sixteen that they had sometimes wished it. These proportions were nearly twice as large as the proportion of young people with two black parents who said they had wished to be another colour. This evidence certainly suggests that mixed parentage is often, although by no means always, experienced in childhood as problematic. Of those who had wished to be another colour, 70 per cent had wished they were white, 10 per cent that they were black, or at least darker than they were, while the remaining 20 per cent wished they were either white or black.

Why should more mixed-parentage than black children want to be another colour? Two factors seemed to be involved: being on the receiving end of abuse from both black and white children, and feeling uncomfortably different from both their black and their white friends. Usually, however, abuse from white children was the sole reason mentioned, as in the following example:

'I went to this [infant] school where there was practically nobody that wasn't white, and from the earliest I can remember that I always got racial abuse ... and the teachers didn't do anything whatsoever about it. I was very ashamed of my colour and I wished I was white. People used to say I was adopted because my mother was white, and stuff. . . . It was really horrible, but when I moved away from that school I discovered that mixed race isn't a problem, it is something to be proud of.'

The small minority who wanted to be black identified strongly with their black parent. The girl quoted below lived with her white mother, but was much more attached to her black father with whom she was in contact. When she was 11 she started to feel she would like to be black. Previously her mother had explained to her that she was like a cup of tea 'a bit of tea, and a bit of milk'.

'I have lived in this house all my life with a load of white people. But they were completely non-racist. And so they didn't even notice that – I mean I knew I was a different colour when I looked in the mirror, but it didn't click to me that meant anything at all. I saw I had a black father and a white mother, so I came out tea-coloured, well, so what, you know . . . and then my dad just said, "Are you black or are you white?" And then I said, "I'm neither, I'm like a cup of tea." And my dad said, "Oh stop this. What are you talking about, you are black. If people see you they are going to think you are black." And I thought, "Oh, that's about it." [*Do you still feel like that?*] No. I have come to the point where I am just glad I am me, you know. I mean, it would be nice if I was just black, but I can't – anyway, I quite like the way I am now.'

The present

The great majority of the mixed-parentage young people – 86 per cent – said, like the girl quoted above, that they did not *now* want to be another colour (Table 6.4). Of those who did, only one said that they often wished this. Of the eight young people concerned, three wanted to be white, one wanted to be black, and four wanted to be either white or black. One of these, who still suffered a good deal of racist abuse, said:

'Sometimes I have sat down and thought, "If I wasn't this colour, I wish I wasn't". It's when people sort of like start talking about my race, and cussing me about it, that's when I sit down and think I wish I wasn't this race and this colouring, but at the end of the day it don't really bother me. [*And which colour have you wished you were?*] I don't know, sometimes it's been white, and sometimes black, it all depends what I'm feeling.'

Another girl, who had a Nigerian father, felt she stood out as different in both countries.

> ''Cos sometimes when I'm in Nigeria these ideas start sparking up
> because I'm always different, always out of it. And also in England,
> if I get called black, 'cos I know that I'm not black, and I'm not
> white, that's when I feel I want to be either, I have no preference
> which I want to be.'

Several of the young people had mixed feelings about their identity. It
was not always clear how troubled they were, but when in doubt we
coded them as wanting to change their colour. One girl, for example,
said:

> 'I often thought, wouldn't it be nice if I could be just one colour, if
> I could be just black or white, but really I wouldn't want to be. . . .
> Sometimes you feel really strongly about it. It's like sometimes you
> think, I wish I wasn't a woman, because of all the situations that
> I'm in, but really, you wouldn't want to change.'

A boy said:

> 'It's not that I've ever actually wished to be white, I'd never, never
> want to be, actually. But there are occasions when you think, if I
> were white, then this wouldn't happen.'

More definite doubts were expressed by another boy:

> 'I'd rather be myself, this colour, and that's true, I would. But I
> think all the time, if I could come back, then I think I would come
> back as a white person, because I'd say it's an easier life.'

There seemed to be several reasons why many of the young people
said they no longer wished to change their colour, though they had
done so in the past. Sometimes acceptance of their colour was triggered
by a single meaningful experience, as in the case of this girl:

> 'Well, when I was little, about 7, I used to [want to be white]
> because the majority of people were white, and I used to think
> white people were a lot prettier. And there was a play in school,
> these people came in and done it, and it was about this black girl
> who wanted to be white, and she got her wish, and she was a

completely ugly white person. And after that I just thought, no, I never want to be white.'

Those who moved to multiracial secondary schools were exposed to widely admired black youth cultures (see Chapter 7). At the same time, they found a larger choice of black, and even mixed-race children, to make friends and form alliances with. The most important factor, however, was probably the development of greater intellectual and emotional maturity. This enabled the young people to cope with racism in ways which had not been available to them earlier (see Chapter 9).

Since only 16 per cent of our mixed-race sample said that they *now* wanted to be another colour, it is not surprising that later in the interview when asked, 'On balance, are you pleased you are mixed race [or half-caste, or whatever label they used]?', 81 per cent said they were, 5 per cent said 'Yes and No', and only one person said she was not. (The remainder said they were just pleased to be themselves, or that colour was irrelevant to them.)

The girl who was not pleased was one of only two young people in our sample to describe the feelings of confusion about her identity traditionally associated with mixed race. (This girl lived with a white parent only, but the boy who expressed confusion lived with both of his parents.)

'Sometimes I feel really confused, as if I don't know in which direction to turn. I feel as if I don't have a true identity, 'cos I've always been brought up with a white community, but then recently I've started to want to understand the black background, and pressure and stuff like that, and sometimes I don't know which one I would call myself, even though generally I think I call myself black.'

When we asked them if they were proud of their mixed parentage, the great majority (77 per cent) said that they were. Later, to a slightly differently worded question, 'How do you feel, now that you are 15 [or whatever age they were] about having one black and one white parent?', about the same proportion (76 per cent) again gave positive answers, and only one young person expressed clearly negative feelings. Of those who gave positive answers, many stressed the advantages of having a foot in both camps.

'They both accept me. Black people don't have to be careful about me, people who are white, they don't have to try and prove that they are not racist, and things like that ... I can go to Notting Hill

Carnival and feel OK and I can go to a very exclusive restaurant where everyone seems to be white, and feel OK . . . I'm pleased that I'm part of each race, yes, I like it.'

[*Are you pleased to be of mixed parentage?*] 'Yes, I'm proud of my colour, you get the best of both worlds. You're not one colour, but two, and I think that's nice.'

'It does mean that I'm comfortable with both white people and black people, which I know a lot of people aren't. And that also I'm accepted by both because I have a white family and a black family.'

Another girl said:

'My mum goes to me, if you have a choice, what would you rather have, two black parents, two white, or would you like it the way it is now? And I always say to her, I like it the way it is now, because I can turn round and say to my mum things I couldn't say to my dad because he's black, and I can turn round and say things to my dad because he's black that I wouldn't like to say to her because it would be hurtful. That's the way I like things to be.'

And another:

'If you look at it superficially, it's a disadvantage, because you are a piggy in the middle, but I think if you look at it deeper it's a definite advantage, because you're not trapped in any group . . . and I think you see things in a clearer perspective, because you're not in the actual centre of the turmoil, you can see things from outside, and you can look at it more objectively.'

While being 'different' from others had been a cause of misery to many in the past, and still was to some, others felt that they benefited from the exoticism of being different.

'I suppose I feel quite special, you know.'

'It's a lot more interesting. If people ask me what nationality I am, I can spend half an hour telling them.' (This girl had a light olive skin.)

'I'm lucky. I'm proud of my colour. [*What makes you proud?*] I'm an individual class, I don't know the word, like we are only a few, sort of thing.'

Others again saw their mixed-race family as a witness against racism.

'I'm glad that my parents are what they are because it shows that people can get on, it doesn't matter what colour they are, people can get on.'

'It's good. It sort of shows that neither family are racist.'

For others, their mixed race was viewed positively because it was part and parcel of their love for their parents, or their own existence.

'Well, I've never known anything different. Well, just like both of my parents, I don't want them to change, I like them as they are.'

'Well, I'm quite glad actually, I'm proud to be born . . . If my mum and dad didn't marry I wouldn't be born, or I'd be born different.'

Only one boy gave an almost wholly negative response. He had expressed mixed feelings when asked earlier whether he was pleased to be of mixed parentage:

'Yes, I'm pleased because I have a better knowledge than most people of both sides. But you have to think of more things, it's harder to relate to people, you've got to analyse their reactions more.'

But when asked later how he felt about his mixed parentage, he gave a more negative response:

'It's hard to relate to parents if one is white and one is black. It's hard for them too, to make a mixed relationship work. It's fine if you know how to deal with it, but I wouldn't like to bring a child of mixed parentage into the world.'

We tried to assess the extent to which our mixed-parentage sample felt positive about their racialised identity by asking two further, more indirect questions. First, we asked if there was any way in which they would like to alter their appearance. Although two-thirds of the sample said that there was, none of their fantasies involved becoming fairer; one girl wanted to be darker and more like her African mother. The most frequently expressed wish was to lose weight. However, nine girls and one boy were dissatisfied with their hair, because it would not grow long and could not be tossed or flicked, while another girl wanted green eyes. Thus about one-fifth of the sample, all but one girls, would have preferred in these respects to look more like a white person. Only four of these eleven showed any other indication of being dissatisfied with their black inheritance.

Later we asked the young people if they would prefer to marry someone of a particular colour, since we thought that a preference for a white or black spouse might indicate that they themselves would like to be that colour. In fact, 75 per cent said they had no colour preference, 13 per cent said they would prefer to marry someone white, and 9 per cent someone mixed race or black, while 3 per cent were not sure.

How many had a positive black identity?

We assessed as having a definitely positive 'racial' identity all those young people who said both that they felt pleased and proud of their mixed parentage, and that, even if in the past they had wanted to be another colour they no longer did so. We excluded from this category anyone who, despite having given these responses, made comments during the course of the interview which suggested they were distressed by feeling 'different', or who seemed to feel confused or anxious or in some other way unhappy about their mixed parentage.

We assessed as having a 'problematic' identity those who said they would still rather be another colour, and/or those whose spontaneous comments indicated that they were unhappy with, or confused about, their mixed parentage. We have labelled this group 'problematic' rather than negative, because all, to a varying extent, expressed contradictory feelings, as in the case of the two girls quoted below.

> 'When I started to mix with boys I just felt different because in my class I'm the only coloured person . . . I felt actually at a disadvantage . . . because everyone's like weighing up what they look like, and I'm different. I think I'll always go through life being a bit different, but sometimes it'll be an advantage as well as a problem . . . I suppose I am pleased I'm neither black nor white, as well as upset because I'm different.'

'Recently I've wanted to be white. [This was in relation to an incident of racialised abuse]. I haven't come across a lot of racial hatred and stuff, but it still hurts you know. I know that if I was white I wouldn't be at all worried about my colour. [*And have you ever thought you would prefer to be black?*] I did about two years ago, I was really into hip hop and hanging around with people who were really rough, and you know sometimes I would get called names by the black people. . . . And then I wished I was black, you know, being in between you can't win either way so you just have to accept it. I like being what I am, because it makes me different, now I like it. But still, I sometimes do wish I was white.'

Later she was fairly positive about her mixed parentage.

'I am happy with the way I am. I mean, I wouldn't say I am proud, but then I can't really see using the word "proud" – unless something happened, then I would be proud. I just think of myself as me.'

Using our fairly stringent criteria, 60 per cent of the sample had a positive racialised identity, and 20 per cent, including the two girls quoted above, had a problematic identity. The remaining 20 per cent, whom we put in the intermediate group, while not wishing to be another colour, were not definitely positive about their racialised identity. In most cases they said, 'it is not a matter of being proud', but some young people whom we put in this group displayed a degree of anxiety centred around their colour. One said:

'Like, I'd see a group of black people walking down the road, say I'm with a white friend, and I always worry, I think, oh, is she going to say something horrible about them, not that she would, it's just that there's a few black people, they're quite rough, and I always worry that they'll be called nasty names, you know, even though they're in the wrong. I just worry sometimes that people get the wrong idea about black people.'

Why did some have a positive identity, and others not?

A positive racialised identity was not associated with coming from a particular social class, or with living in a family with a black parent, or with thinking of oneself as black. Nearly three-quarters of those with a positive identity thought of themselves as 'mixed', or brown, or, in one case, usually as white. Since this girl did in fact look white, but made no attempt to conceal her parentage and was proud of it, we thought it reasonable to say that she had a positive racialised identity.

There was a statistically significant tendency for those who currently wished to be another colour to be strongly affiliated to white people (Table 6.5: see Appendix). There was a tendency, which approached statistical significance, for those with a positive identity to attend multiracial schools (Table 6.6: see Appendix). And there was a stronger, and statistically significant tendency, for those who had a *problematic* identity to say they had been told by their parents to be proud of being black, or of being of mixed parentage. Of the young people with a positive identity, only 38 per cent said they had been told this, as did 36 per cent of those with an intermediate identity, compared with 82 per cent of those with a problematic identity. The most likely explanation of this counter-intuitive finding seems to us to be that the parents of the young people with a problematic identity sensed they were lacking in confidence, or anxious about themselves, or about their colour, specifically. In response to these perceptions the parents attempted to boost their morale by telling them they should be proud of their colour. One girl's comment suggests that this had happened in her case.

> 'Yes [she had been told to be proud] but that is when I get a bit sort of upset. Like when I came back from the party [where racist remarks had been made to her] and my mum said "You should be proud of what you are, you are a lovely colour" and all that sort of stuff. It makes me feel better now, it didn't when I was younger.'

Of the three pairs of siblings in the sample, each member of the pair differed from the other in the degree to which they had a positive identity. The differences might have been due to differences in the extent to which they worried or were lacking in confidence. However, their relationships with one or other parent were not equally positive, and it seems possible that this influenced how positive they felt about their racialised identity. (These last two factors may well be related.)

How central was their racialised identity to the lives of the young people?

An identity which is central is easily activated, aroused by even minimal cues in the environment, so that one is frequently aware of it. One way of assessing the centrality of an identity is therefore to ask how much time is spent thinking about it. Only five of the young people said that their mixed parentage was always, or nearly always, on their mind. They appeared to be preoccupied by it in a very negative sense. They were all at predominantly white schools, and all but one were assessed by us as having a problematic racialised identity.

> 'I suppose it's on my mind most of the time. [*Why is that?*] I worry that people will discriminate against me because of my colour, and being aware that I'm the only coloured person in my class.'

> 'Yes, I'm always aware of it. Whenever I'm in a black community, I'm always aware of it because I'm slightly different, and also when I'm in a white community. And also, I'm always conscious when I meet new people in case they're going to be racist.'

On the other hand, 37 per cent of the sample said they hardly ever thought about their colour. A typical comment was: 'In this [school] environment, where no one's racist, you don't really think about it.'

The largest group of the young people, 54 per cent, said they were sometimes conscious of their mixed parentage, but not very often. Going into the country was one situation which was often cited as bringing it to consciousness. Thus one girl said:

> 'In the country, or in cities where there aren't a lot of black people, if you go there, it's nudge, wink, look, over there's a black person, as if they'd never seen one before, but when you come back to London, it's like nobody cares whether you're black or white.'

Other situations which made them aware of their colour included being asked where their parents came from, hearing racist remarks or disputes about race, and going to unfamiliar discos and clubs.

There is another sense in which an identity can be central, which is concerned not with the amount of time one is aware of it, but with its tendency to be an organising principle in one's mind, to which other matters are referred. (In this sense gender is very central to feminists.) We attempted to assess the centrality of the young people's racialised identity in this sense in the final question of our interview. We gave them cards, on each of which was written one of the eleven topics discussed in the interview (their family, friends, education, gender, colour, social class, nationality, etc.). We asked them to rank in order the seven most important topics for their sense of identity, which we defined as 'the sense of who you are', and to discard any that were not important to their identity. One-third of the young people put colour among their first four choices, while 39 per cent did not include it at all. One of these, who looked white, said:

'I don't think colour is part of my identity, I never really thought of myself before this interview as any colour. But that doesn't necessarily mean that I don't have a sense of identity. [*What do you mean by saying that colour doesn't form part of your identity?*] Well, I think it does, but for me it doesn't matter, I don't feel, oh God, I don't belong, or anything.'

As well as asking this direct question, we explored the extent to which the young people believed that their mixed parentage impinged on a variety of aspects of their lives. These included whether they thought their school experiences would have been different if they had more black teachers – 48 per cent thought they would. One reason often given was that they believed black teachers would have a greater understanding of how racist abuse affected them.

'I think in some situations they would have been more understanding, like a couple of kids can be really racist in class, and you get really angry and het up about it, and an argument can start up easily, and the teachers don't understand why you get so angry. Black teachers would understand exactly, because they would know, maybe have had those experiences before.'

Others thought white teachers were not strict enough with black children.

'A lot of the black kids get away with it when they go to a school where it's all white teachers . . . say a black boy has had a fight, and he had broken someone's ribs or something. A lot of teachers would think, oh well I've heard his mother's really rough, and she knows how to give you a mouthful . . . we can't suspend him because his mother's going to come up. . . . When you've got black teachers, it's more stricter, 'cos they are trying to teach you not to do wrong, they are trying to lead you, you know, in the right direction.'

An equal number of young people did not see colour as of central importance in relation to teachers; what mattered was whether they taught well. In fact, only half of the young people of mixed parentage had been taught by a black teacher, compared to 70 per cent of those with two black parents, a difference which reflects the larger proportion of the mixed-parentage sample in independent schools.

Other questions on centrality included whether they thought their lives so far would have been more difficult if they had two black parents – 34 per cent thought they would; or in the future – 43 per cent thought so; or if they thought their lives in the future would be easier if they were white – 50 per cent thought so.

Finally, we asked them if they would prefer to live in a mainly white, or mainly black, or a mixed neighbourhood. If colour was of little significance in their lives, one might expect them to say they had no preference. In fact, only 21 per cent did so. The majority (68 per cent) opted for a mixed area, with the remaining 11 per cent divided between those who would prefer a white area and those who would prefer a black area.

For which young people was colour most central?

Combining the answers to these questions on centrality as an organising principle into a score from 0 to 8, we found no relationship between the combined score and most 'background' factors, such as social class, gender, or type of school. There was, however, a significant relationship with the racialised mix of the family (Table 6.7: see Appendix). One-fifth of the sample for whom race was *least* central were all living with one or two black parents, but had little contact with other black people. Those for whom race was *most* central tended to be more affiliated to black people, to feel most comfortable with others of mixed parentage, and to have had more personal experience of racism.

Summary and discussion

Less than half of our sample thought of themselves as black. Most of the rest had a 'mixed' or 'brown' identity, a small number thinking of themselves as 'more white than black'. Although we classified them according to their answers to the direct questions about identity, other comments they made suggested that their racialised identities did not always fit neatly into these categories. As the above quotations illustrate, some seemed to switch backwards and forwards between identifications in the course of the interview, while others described themselves as having a different racialised identity in different situations.

Defining one's identity as black was not related to social class, or the racialised composition of the family or school. It *was* related to holding more politicised ideas about racism. In addition, those young people who looked white tended not to think of themselves as black.

Some of the young people were unwilling to identify themselves as black because of their loyalty to, and identification with, one or other or both of their parents. When we asked them which side they would take in a hypothetical conflict between black and white people, 41 per cent chose the black side, and 13 per cent the white. However, 38 per cent refused to choose, often saying, as did this girl, 'Well, I'd be alienating one of my parents if I chose, and I wouldn't like to do that.'

It is these familial ties which for many make their situation, and hence their identity, different from that of young people with two black parents. They resisted pressure to be either black or white, because they felt themselves to be *both*. Even if they were seen as black by others, they *experienced* themselves as 'mixed'.

This sense of dual loyalties is central to the concept of 'marginality' (see Chapter 3). However, while it was assumed by the marginality theorists that marginality is inherently painful and accompanied by a confused or negative identity, only a minority of our sample approximated to this description. While half of the sample had in the past wished to be another colour, the great majority no longer did so. Most said they were proud of their mixed parentage. We assessed 60 per cent as having a definitely positive racialised identity, 20 per cent as having a problematic one, and 20 per cent as intermediate. Only two of the young people appeared to feel confused about their racialised identity.

But although the majority had a positive identity, the proportion who wished they were another colour was twice as large as in the group with two black parents. It is still not an easy ride to be of mixed black and white parentage in our society – because of racism, the situation is very different from that of, say, children with one British and one French parent. It is also more difficult in some respects from that of young people with two black parents, partly because some meet hostility both from black and white people (see Chapter 8), and partly because some feel 'different' from both. Difference is not in itself a negative characteristic – some young people regarded their difference as interesting or exotic – but it can be so if it is defined by others as negative. Nevertheless, the majority of the young people were able to regard their mixed parentage as an asset, to a degree that was probably not possible in the past. Factors likely to have contributed to this change include altered societal attitudes to mixed marriages (Chapter 2), the rise of black youth cultures, much admired by sectors of white youth (Chapter 7), and the antiracist ethos in some London schools (Chapter 8).

Why did some have a positive racialised identity, while others did not? Unexpectedly, the parental strategy of telling their children to be proud of their colour was more frequently reported by young people with a problematic identity, presumably because they seemed to their parents to be more in need of reassurance. We found a not very strong relationship between having a positive identity and attending a multi-racial school, and a much stronger one between currently wishing they were another colour, and the strength of their affiliation to white people. Because siblings differed in their racialised identities, we suspect, also, that family dynamics and the self-esteem of the young people are influences on whether their racialised identity is positive. Having a positive racialised identity was *not* associated with living with a black parent.

We found the 'racial' terms attacked by some black people since the 1960s – particularly 'coloured' and 'half-caste' – still widely used by black, white and mixed-parentage young people. Those from working-class families, and those of our mixed-parentage sample with less politicised views of racism, were most likely to use them. Colour was much more central in the lives of some young people than in others. Those for whom colour was most central tended to be those with more experience of racism, and more black friends, and those who said they felt most comfortable with other people of mixed parentage. Those for whom colour was least central were more often living with black, rather than only white, parents. This seemed to be because a number of black parents and mixed couples in our sample lived in white suburbs and sent their children to predominantly white independent schools, so that they knew few, if any, young black people.

Contrary to much current theorising, we found then, no evidence that having a black identity, or a positive racialised identity, or a racialised identity that was very central, were associated with living with a black parent. But these aspects of their racialised identities *were* related to the extent to which the young people held politicised views about racism, and were strongly affiliated to white people. Whether living with a black parent is necessary in order to acquire 'survival skills' in a racist society, and 'black culture and attitudes', are topics we explore in the next three chapters.

7   Friendships and allegiances

In a non-racist society, mixed black and white parentage, like mixed British and French parentage, might be seen as a definite advantage, allowing insights and an entree into both groups. The situation is likely to be different when one group is less powerful, and is considered inferior by the other. Then, according to the marginality theorists (Chapter 3) people of mixed parentage will inevitably be social isolates, distrusted and rejected by both groups. A rather different concern, expressed by social workers, is that mixed-parentage children reared in white families will be unable to relate to black people and to black culture. On the other hand, some of the young people in our study told us that one of the advantages of being of mixed parentage was the ability to bridge both cultures, and to feel at ease with both white and black people. In this chapter we discuss the extent to which these opposing claims are supported by evidence from our interviews about the young people's friendships, cultural allegiances and loyalties.

Comfort with black and white people

In answer to the direct question 'Do you feel more comfortable with black or with white people?' one-third of the sample said that at times they felt some discomfort with one or other group. Slightly more of these young people said they felt uncomfortable with black people than those who said they felt uncomfortable with white.

Unexpectedly, all those who said they felt more comfortable with white people than with black lived with one or two black parents. The explanation for this finding seemed to lie in part in the fact that many of these parents sent their children to independent, almost entirely white schools. Consequently they had few, if any, black friends. It seemed that living with a black parent was not enough to give them a feeling of ease with black people if, as was sometimes the case, their parent was the only black person whom they knew well. One such girl, all of whose friends were white, said:

> 'I'm more comfortable with white people, 'cos I'm used to them more. I've never been in, sort of, in a group of totally black people, ever.'

Another said:

> 'I mean, the only time I have ever actually been with any coloured people that are really black is through my [African] mother, and usually they are people that I don't know, so I feel more comfortable with white people.'

Several young people from middle-class families, both boys and girls, were uneasy with young black males, rather than black people in general. The girl quoted below, who lived with her black middle-class mother and a white step-parent, had no black friends. Her fear of black men was, as she admitted, not related to her own experience, but probably derived from the media.

> 'I am not prejudiced against any race at all, except, I don't know what it is, but when I am walking down the street say dead at night, I feel threatened when I see a bunch of black men rather than white men, but that is as far as my prejudice – I mean, I wouldn't call it prejudice, I am just wary of that. [*Why do you think that is?*] It could be propaganda from the newspapers, I mean, the sort of picture they build up is that a lot of street crimes are from black men. Also I get a lot of wolf-whistles and they generally tend to be from black men, and I find there is this hostility from black men to women that I don't like. It is something that I feel more with black young men in hip hop gear, I mean if he was in a suit, I suppose actually I don't mean black men in general, it's the way they dress.'

A boy who lived with his black mother and attended a predominantly white independent school had similar, probably media-induced, fears.

> [*Do you feel more comfortable with white or black people?*] 'It depends on whether I know them well. If I don't know them I'm wary of black kids, raggas, of being mugged by black people.'

However, discomfort with black people was not always due to

unfamiliarity with them. There were instances where, despite attending a multiracial school and living with both parents in a multiracial area, young people, like the boy quoted below, felt more at ease with white people.

'With black people I'm sometimes worried whether they're seeing me, looking at me and thinking, he thinks he's black, doesn't he, but I know white people never ever think like that . . . they just sort of, like, see me.

'Like my friends, sometimes they forget what my colour is, and they just see me as a white person, but that doesn't offend me.'

This boy's uneasy relationship with black youth, and identification with his white friends, emerged in the following account, in which it becomes clear that he regards mugging as a racial crime. ('They didn't want my money, because I was their own colour.')

'I was with my [white] friends in Macdonalds, and these black kids came in to mug, to get money off my friends. They never had no money to give them, so out of politeness, because I didn't want no trouble, I gave them my money, I said "Look, you can take some of this". Like I didn't give them all of it, just a pound, and they went, "No, it's all right, we don't want your money". So I goes, "It's the same colour as theirs", and they took it, and then they just went and bought a hamburger, actually. So I told my mum, and she said I shouldn't have given them money, because the next time they see me in the street they'll think, oh yes, we'll get money off him, but I don't think my mum understood, they didn't want my money, because I was their own colour. But my dad was quite angry with me giving the money, because he said that's low. They were going round sort of like forcibly begging off people, and they shouldn't do that.'

Six of the fifty-eight young people said they felt uncomfortable with white people. Paradoxically again, three lived in an all-white family. Despite having some white friends, they felt more relaxed with black people.

'If I'm with a group of white people that I don't know, and they are all white and I'm the only black person there, then I feel that they might be looking down on me, or noticing me especially. Whereas if you are in a group of black people, they are used to seeing a black person's face, and if they are looking at you it's just 'cos of what you are, not what your colour is.'

Another girl, who lived with both parents, was closely attached to her white mother, and did not regard herself as black. Nevertheless, she had mainly black friends and felt more comfortable with black people.

'I think I'm more comfortable with black people, I must admit. [*Why?*] 'Cos I share the same culture and music, things like that, food, clothing, I suppose. [*So food, even though your mother's white?*] Yes, she cooks like a West Indian, my mum does.'

The girl quoted earlier, who was frightened of black men, was balanced by the boy quoted below, who felt threatened by white people he did not know.

'In quite a few places sometimes I feel safer being around black people than I do being around a load of white people . . . like on the Tube, if it was like full of white people . . . but I don't really notice it that much here' [at school].

Since, as we noted in Chapter 6, some of the young people in the sample were uncomfortably aware of feeling 'different' from both black and white people, we went on to ask, 'Do you feel most comfortable with people of mixed race?' One-third of the sample said they did, although some commented that they knew very few.

'Yes, I think so, because you can always talk about what problems you have, and they understand how you feel.'

'Yes, they really understand how it feels. Sometimes you feel you're piggy in the middle, and I think all in all I feel most comfortable with mixed-race people.'

Another girl, who had both black and white friends, but none of mixed parentage, had a great desire to know others like herself.

'Yes, yes, I would. I was saying to my friend the other day, I wonder what it would be like to go to an all half-caste school. I was just thinking how it would be. And my mum was saying to me, would I feel better, and I goes, No, I won't feel no different, I would just like to experience it to see what it was like, and see if every other half-caste person was just like me. 'Cos everyone says I'm loud and outgoing, and I just think – I wonder if they are all like me or if they are really quiet, you know.'

Young people from working-class families, and those attending multiracial schools, and state schools, were significantly more likely to say that they felt more comfortable with others of mixed parentage, perhaps because they were more likely to know some, or perhaps because they were more likely to have met discrimination from both black and white young people (Table 7.1: see Appendix).

Negative feelings towards black and white people

About a quarter of the sample felt not necessarily uncomfortable with, but negative towards, either black or white people. When we asked, 'What do you feel about black people generally?' and 'What do you feel about white people generally?' 13 per cent gave negative answers about black people, and 11 per cent about white. One girl said:

'At the end of the day, I think they [white people] will always feel superior, even if they don't acknowledge it, even if it's a sort of subconscious feeling, because they've always been in the majority. If I sat down with a friend, you know, my best friend is white, and we listened to something and it was racist, she might not pick up on it, but I would, I don't know, it's just something about them. You know they will be saying, Oh yes, of course I get on with you, but you've still got the feeling that at the end of the day they're thinking, well, you know, she's still black.'

Another was critical of the older generation of African Caribbeans.

'I think some of them can be quite old-fashioned, and have very Victorian attitudes. Some of the people that come from the West Indies, definitely. The men are quite chauvinistic, some of them.'

Of those who made negative remarks about black people, all but one lived with a black parent, as did all but one of those who made negative remarks about white people. We suspected, although we had no systematic evidence on this point, that the negative remarks were related to a poor relationship with a parent of that colour.

These young people were, however, very much in the minority. The boy quoted below gave a much more typical response:

'When I look at someone and they're black I don't say, Oh that person's black, so I'm gonna think this about him, I just wait and see what that person is. I don't treat anyone differently because of their colour.'

Answers of this kind (that one cannot generalise from colour) or positive comments were given by three-quarters of the sample. And, as described above, two-thirds of the sample said they felt equally comfortable with both black and white people.

Neighbourhood preference

A preference for living in a mainly white or mainly black area could be considered an indicator of 'racial' allegiance. However, only a very small proportion of the sample (8 per cent) said they would prefer a white neighbourhood, and 4 per cent a black neighbourhood. The great majority of mixed-parentage young people said either that they would prefer to live in a racially mixed area (68 per cent) or that they did not mind what kind of neighbourhood they lived in (19 per cent). Preference for a mixed area at times seemed to be an affirmation of their mixed status; at other times it reflected an anxiety about racism.

'You hear of people who live in all-white areas, they get a bit of hassle. Maybe it is not as bad as it sounds, but I worry about that sort of thing. I feel more comfortable if I see somebody of mixed race or whatever around, so I would feel I don't mind turning my music up loud. If it was all white people in the street, I definitely wouldn't want to live there.'

Those who wanted to live in a white neighbourhood had fears about black masculinity, like this girl, who accepted the widely held stereotype of black men.

'I'd prefer a white neighbourhood, because I feel more secure when I'm with white people, I know it sounds bad, but I do. [*Secure in what way?*] Well, like with our area, you don't want to walk the streets anywhere, not even in the daytime, I don't feel safe, because there's always black guys hanging round, and they make the place look so untidy, they whistle at you and say horrible things. I just can't stand it, and white people are not like that I don't think, in, you know, upper-class areas.'

Social class and colour preference were in conflict for a number of the young people from middle-class families, because of their unease with working-class black people. One girl expressed the conflict as follows:

'I would quite like to live in Brixton [a mainly working-class area with a higher proportion of black people than most]. At least it's got atmosphere, it's got an identity. I would also like to walk around and be in the majority, the black people, I think it would be a laugh, you know.' However, she went on to say: 'But having been to a private school, I would rather live in a middle-class area, really . . . and that's a bit contradictory, isn't it. If I want to live in a middle-class area that would mean living in a white area, is that true? Of course there are middle-class black people, but I'm not sure if they live in the same area as middle-class white people.'

Friends

Friends were very important in the lives of the young people we interviewed. When we asked at the end of the interview which of the various topics we had discussed were the most important to their identity – that is, their sense of who they were – half put friends as their first or second choice, second only to their families. One girl said:

'I can talk to my friends about things I can't really talk to my parents about, because well – they seem to understand me more, and my parents don't really always listen to me, and my friends do, because they've been in the same situations as me.'

The young people often used the term 'friend' in quite a loose sense, to refer to young people whom they 'hung around with'. Some numbered as many as sixty friends at school, and fifty out of school. Only 16 per cent said they had fewer than five friends at school.

One boy at an independent school said:

'I mix with a lot of people at school, 'cos I do a lot of activities and have a lot of friends. I just don't make enemies, really, I have a lot of people I get on well with, probably about thirty. [*And out of school?*] There's a small group I associate with most of the time, about ten, mainly boys, and it enlarges to about fifty, about half boys and half girls.'

However, they all accepted a distinction between friends and close friends. The boy quoted above, for example, said he had four close friends, all boys, while the girl whose views on the importance of friends were quoted earlier said she had 'loads' of friends out of school, different groups of friends, but only about four or five close friends, all girls, who were 'in and out of' her house. Only one person said they had no close friends.

Usually school and out-of-school friends overlapped, but for a quarter of the sample they were completely separate.

> 'My friends in school, they don't really listen to acid [acid house music] or nothing, whereas out of school I've got two friends – one white girl and one black girl – and like all of us are totally into acid, a day won't go past when we're not, you know, dressed up in the clothes what tell people that you listen to acid, whereas friends in school, they just sort of dress in jeans and jumpers and track suits. [*And are they the only friends that you hang around with out of school?*] Well, there's a bunch of boys, right, well, we're not really with them, sort of half the time we are, if we're not doing nothing we might go in the park and sit down and have a laugh, like, and the bunch of boys will come over as well.'

Although two-thirds of the mixed-parentage group said they felt equally comfortable with black and white people, their friends were more often white than black. While 85 per cent had a close white friend, only 42 per cent had a close black friend, and only 30 per cent had both. A sizeable minority (27 per cent) had no black friends, either in or out of school. With one exception, all the young people without black friends attended independent schools, and lived in almost entirely white areas. In contrast, only one person in the sample had no white friends. This was a girl who said that her black father had advised her not to trust white people. She said that she disliked white people, and found it difficult to talk freely to them.

Selection of friends depends not only on attraction but on opportunity, and it cannot be assumed that young people with no black or mixed-parentage friends do not want them. Rather, over half our sample attended predominantly white schools, and many lived in white areas, so it was not surprising to find that half had no black friends at school, and that under half had a close black friend. In a similar way, the possibility of someone in our sample having a friend who was of mixed parentage was limited by the scarcity of young people of mixed parentage. Only 18 per cent had a close friend who was of mixed parentage.

Boyfriends, girlfriends and marriage partners

We asked the young people about the colour of their current and past boyfriends or girlfriends. Twelve per cent of the mixed-parentage sample said they had never had one, but for the rest, their boyfriends or girlfriends, like other friends, had more often been white (78 per cent of cases) than black (44 per cent). Thirty per cent of the young people said they had both white and black boyfriends or girlfriends. Half this number (15 per cent) had been out with an Asian boy or girl, while even fewer (8 per cent) had been out with a boy or girl of mixed parentage.

That the preponderance of white girlfriends and boyfriends was generally a matter of availability rather than preference is suggested by the finding that a large majority – three-quarters of the sample – said they had no colour preference for a marriage partner. Thirteen per cent said they would prefer to marry, or live with, someone white, 4 per cent someone of mixed parentage, and 8 per cent someone either black or of mixed parentage. An example of the most frequent response to our question came from a girl whose boyfriends had all been black:

'I don't care what colour I marry. It's not, colour doesn't matter, as long as they're decent people, you know.'

Another girl, who had both black and white boyfriends, said:

'Well, I'm in two minds. I think if I married a white person, then the kid would turn out quite stunning if they had blue eyes, 'cos I'm completely in love with half-caste children with blue eyes – the kid would probably have brown eyes anyway, knowing my luck. But ideally I think it should be a black person. [*Why do you think it's ideal?*] I think it is a more stable relationship. I think if I married a white person, if I had an argument with him, I would probably say, oh yes, who do you think you are talking to, some ignorant nigger, I would probably throw that at him, which really doesn't show a lot of trust for your partner.'

Those who opted for another person of mixed parentage tended to have the appearance of their children in mind.

'Only because of how my kids would turn out, I suppose I'd like them to be as close to my colour as possible.'

A preference for a white partner was usually explained in terms of finding white people more attractive or being more used to them. The girl quoted below lived with her African mother, but looked white, went to an almost exclusively white school, and had no black friends.

'Whenever I think of myself as married, I never see myself married to a coloured person . . . I don't think I'm prejudiced against black people, I don't know why it is. [*So you think you're much more likely to marry someone white?*] Yes. [*Have you got a reason why that would be?*] I don't know, it's probably cos I don't really know that many black people.'

Another girl, who was quite dark skinned, and lived with a black mother, but who again knew very few black people, had clearly incorporated white standards of beauty:

'If I fell in love with someone of any colour then I would marry him. But I think, judging from my life now, it's more likely that I will marry a white man, because most of my friends are, and I find white men more attractive than any other.'

Heroes and heroines

As another indicator of alignment with black or white people, we asked the young people whether they had any heroes or heroines, people whom they admired very much. Sixty-three per cent said that they had, as did 62 per cent of the black group, but only 40 per cent of the white group. The greater proportion of young people in the black and mixed-parentage groups having heroes or heroines was almost entirely due to the fact that a substantial proportion of them (30 per cent in the case of the mixed-parentage group, and 49 per cent in the case of the black group) named a political leader, generally Nelson Mandela or Martin Luther King. In contrast, only 8 per cent of young white people named either a black or a white political leader (almost always Margaret Thatcher). But about the same proportion of black, white and mixed-parentage young people named heroes or heroines from the music and film world, and from sport. In the case of the mixed-parentage group, they were equally likely to be black or white.

Which young people were more affiliated to black people, and which to white?

We gave each of the young people two scores on the basis of their answers to the questions on the colour of their friends, whether they were more comfortable with black or white people, their colour preference for a future partner, and for an area to live in, and whether they named black or white heroes and heroines. The scores were a measure of the strength of their affiliation to white and to black people. There were very significant relationships between attending multiracial and state schools, believing their parents had influenced their views on racism, and affiliation to black people, and between attending predominantly white and independent schools, believing their parents had *not* influenced their views, and affiliation to white people (Tables 7.2 and 7.3: see Appendix). Living with white parents only was significantly related to being affiliated to black people, while living with black parents only was significantly related to being affiliated to white people, a finding which seemed related to the tendency of many black parents in our sample to send their children to predominantly white schools.

Allegiance to black youth cultures

Flourishing black youth cultures have developed in Britain in the past thirty years, focused on new forms of music, most of which are a fusion of influences from the Caribbean and the USA (Gilroy, 1987: 192). Each type of music has its own subculture, with its own ideology and distinctive style of dress, attracting a different sector of youth, who listen to different radio stations, and go to parties and clubs where they meet other fans and hear their favourite kind of music. Since these subcultures are constantly feeding off each other and changing, it might be more appropriate to refer to them as 'styles'. Black music was the favourite music of half of the mixed-parentage young people, a quarter of the white sample, and 83 per cent of the black sample. The kinds of black music they liked, in descending order of preference, were soul, hip hop, reggae, ragga, jazz and house music. A few mentioned funk and blues, but no one mentioned calypso or gospel. Ragga music, which has a wide following among London youth, has two kinds of lyrics: one which incorporates boasting, and another which is concerned with the plight of young black people in England.

Admirers of these different music forms tend to adopt different styles of dress. In the hip hop style, clothes tend to be loose and baggy, and caps, gold chains and 'trainers' of specific (expensive) makes, with very thick soles and enormous tongues, are worn. Ragga adherents, called raggamuffins, tend to be younger. They use a black London argot, go round in a 'posse', and are reputed to be aggressive. One mixed-parentage boy in our sample was a raggamuffin, as were or had been three girls, two of whom came from middle-class families, but had some black working-class friends. However, one of the girls had just stopped being ragga, and the other was not fully committed. This girl said:

> 'I like dressing raggamuffin, I feel more comfortable, more confident dressed like this, because you know that nobody is going to come up and mess you about, because they are all scared of you. . . . You can just scare the hell out of most people.'

However, she was critical of raggamuffins who could not change styles.

> 'I think it's a bit sad when all the raggamuffin people, they look nice in that sort of style, but if you ask them to change it, to go out dressed smart, they can't get it together, they can only stick to one thing. Which I think, you know, people ought to be a bit more versatile.'

The other girl had recently abandoned her allegiance because of the way of life of the raggas she knew.

> 'It's your big clumpy trainers, and your gold chains, your caps, your leather, all that type of thing, you know, smoking drugs. You walk down the street, OK, and people used to look at you as if to say, oh God, I'd better keep out of your way, people of your own age who are not identified with that image. I mean, don't get me, it's not all black or mixed race or Asian, there are a few white youths who associate with it, as well . . . it's very much against the police and against the system. . . . When I started to think, well what am I doing here? was when people [raggamuffins] started going round stealing things, shoplifting, you know, attacking people. There was one girl I know, I'm not going to say her name, and this ragga boy said something to her, and she cheeked him back, and he punched her, she's got this big black eye at the moment. It's so aggressive that I just don't want to associate with it.'

At the time of our study acid house followers tended to wear bright colours, floral patterns and have a generally 'hippy' appearance, while adherents of soul and jazz, often older, preferred to dress in a smart, even flashy style. However, these generalisations should be treated with caution. Like other fashions, black youth fashions are constantly changing, and the styles worn by girls are often rather different from those worn by boys. In our study, black youth clothes styles were worn by less than half of those who admired the music – by 41 per cent of the black sample, 20 per cent of those of mixed parentage, and only 4 per cent of the white sample.

Both clothes and hairstyles, as the young people we interviewed were well aware, make a definite statement about the wearer's identity, and facilitate group solidarity. This is equally true of speech styles, which in our sample ranged from black London and black Caribbean styles to white middle-class standard English. Unfortunately, we did not assess either speech styles or hairstyles, both important aspects of black youth culture; the former would have been a very time-consuming task.

Only half of the mixed-parentage group said they preferred black music. Of the rest, 20 per cent said they liked 'most kinds of music', and another 20 per cent liked pop music best. Although pop music has black exponents, it was acknowledged by the young people in our sample to be 'white' music, as was rock and classical music. Only 4 per cent liked classical music best, and only 4 per cent rock, which was the favourite music of a quarter of the white sample, but none of the black.

Whilst only one-fifth of the mixed-parentage sample dressed in a black youth style, clothes styles were of concern to the majority. Only one-third said they did not dress in any particular style. Most of those who did not dress in a black style said they followed the fashions, or that they had developed their own style.

Those who admired black music did not always dress in a black youth style, or preferentially listen to black radio stations. Certain 'black' radio stations, including both legal stations (such as Choice FM) and pirate stations (such as Fantasy and Centre Force), form an important part of black youth culture; some young people in the sample never listened to mainstream radio. Their favourite stations were almost entirely given over to playing recorded music, each station specialising in one type of music. These black radio stations were the favourite stations of 61 per cent of the black sample, but of only 27 per cent of the mixed-parentage sample; most of the rest preferred Capital Radio (40 per cent), Radio 1 (9 per cent) or Radio 4 (7 per cent).

Which young people were attracted to black youth cultures?

We gave each of the young people a score of 0 to 3 for their allegiance to black youth cultures, depending on whether they expressed a preference for black youth music, black youth fashions and black radio stations. Forty-three per cent had a score of 0; that is, they shared none of these tastes. Those with the strongest allegiance to black youth culture were significantly more often those who attended multiracial and state schools, and came from working-class families (Table 7.4: see Appendix).

Some of the young people were very well aware of this association, either because of their fear of young black males, whom they saw as embodiments of black youth cultures, or, as in the case of the girl quoted below, because they resented the annexation of 'blackness' by adherents of black youth cultures.

> 'And he [a black boy] turned round and said, Oh, what's the matter, are we too black for you? And I just thought that was a really ignorant thing to say, because what defines blackness, there isn't anything, you know. I could say, OK, I've lived in Africa for two years, and you haven't even been there. . . . And I thought, so I've gone to quite a posh school, and I speak the English language properly, does that mean that I'm not black? Do you have to go round wearing baggy trousers and trainers and drop your t's to be black? I mean, I can do that quite well, as it goes. When I go out you wouldn't know that I went to a private school, but I wouldn't say that's being black . . . if they say that if you've got a good accent, then you're trying to be white, then that means that you have to run around saying "All right man, how's it going". Why can't black people speak the English language properly? Oh, it's stupid.'

Links with African Caribbean culture

All the young people in our sample had grown up in a culture very different from the African or African Caribbean culture in which one of their parents had been reared. Although half of them had some allegiance to contemporary black youth cultures, these tend to have their roots in the USA as well as in the Caribbean. We felt uncertain about the extent to which our mixed-parentage sample would identify with their African or Caribbean roots. More particularly, those mixed-parentage young people reared by white parents might be expected to have few links with the cultures of their black parent.

Belonging to a culture includes not only sharing a language, religion, music, arts and customs, aspects which are relatively easy to assess, but also sharing values and having a feeling of a shared past and of identification with the cultures. These are difficult issues to explore and assess quantitatively, as we discovered in our pilot study. In the end we decided to focus on food preferences, which are usually a deeply rooted aspect of cultures, interest in black magazines and newspapers with Caribbean links, religion, and indications of loyalty to their black parent's country. ·

Among the mixed-parentage group, two-thirds said they liked African or Caribbean food and two-thirds British food; 40 per cent liked both. Almost as many (62 per cent) liked Chinese food, followed by Italian and Greek (57 per cent), while Indian food was the least popular, liked by only 46 per cent of the sample. This ranking of food preferences was the same in both the black and white groups, except that many more of the young black people (89 per cent) and many fewer of the white (10 per cent) liked African or Caribbean food.

Liking African or Caribbean food was significantly associated with coming from a working-class family and attending a multiracial school (Table 7.5: see Appendix). Surprisingly, it was not related to living with a black parent – an equal proportion of those living only with white people did so. In their case, the young people had either eaten such food with black friends or relations, or their mother had learned how to cook it when living with her black partner.

Few of the young people of mixed parentage showed much interest in the black media, except in relation to black youth cultures. Only 7 per cent of the mixed-parentage group, compared with 31 per cent of the black group, read black magazines or newspapers, usually *Ebony*, *The Voice*, and the *Gleaner*. Even in these instances the young people did not buy the papers themselves, but read them if a parent or sibling bought them. The girls usually bought *Just Seventeen*, *Elle* and *Looks*; the boys, video or pop magazines (such as Sky) or sports, car or computer magazines. In discussing their favourite TV programmes, only 13 per cent mentioned programmes featuring black people or black issues, compared with 34 per cent of the black group. (There are, of course, very few such programmes available.) In all but one case the programme mentioned was *The Cosby Show*, a soap opera about a middle-class American black family. The exception was a boy who looked out for programmes dealing with racism. Much the most popular TV programmes were soaps, especially the Australian soaps, *Neighbours* and *Home and Away.*

Loyalty to African Caribbean or African origins

Over half (57 per cent) of the mixed-parentage sample had made one or more visits to their black parent's country of origin, so to them, at least, it was not an abstract concept. Most spoke enthusiastically about their visits, although some who had visited African countries had been offended by encounters with sexism and anti-white sentiments. However, in virtually all cases the experience had been little more than a pleasant holiday, and they had not been tempted to settle there.

> 'I love Trinidad, I enjoy it as a holiday place, but I wouldn't want to live there. I don't consider myself Trinidadian, I'm English.'

> 'I stayed there for like a month and a half, and I didn't take to it, I had to leave because it was just so small. If I was going to settle anywhere else it would have to be in a big city.'

Only three of the mixed-parentage sample, none of whom had visited the Caribbean, considered living there a possibility. (No one said they wanted to live in an African country.)

> 'I don't know, it depends. If I go to Jamaica and like it, I think I'll stay there, or if I went to America and I liked it, I might live there, but it depends if I thought my family would come. I can't take it to live far away from my mum.'

While 57 per cent thought they would probably live most of their lives in England, and 7 per cent did not know, 36 per cent said they would like to settle in another country. The black group were even more adventurous in their plans, the white group rather less so.

For all groups, the USA was most frequently mentioned as a place to move to, and seen as a land of opportunity and excitement.

> 'I want to go and live in the States – if I can work things out then I would stay, so long as I made a lot of money so I could travel back and forth, because you know I have strong family ties, so I don't think I could live without seeing my mum for a year. [*Why the States?*] Because it's so different – everything is like so much bigger there.'

We know from studies of second-generation Irish in Britain that thinking of themselves as Irish, or half Irish, is strongly linked with retaining other aspects of Irish identity (Ullah, 1985). Similar studies have been carried out with Mexican Americans in the USA (Lampe, 1978). When we asked the young people in our sample whether they thought of themselves as English or British or neither, only 7 per cent of the mixed-parentage sample, all of whom had lived for some time in an African country, said they thought of themselves as Kenyan, Nigerian, etc. Another 14 per cent thought of themselves as half British and half Caribbean or African; half of these young people had been born in Africa.

However, not all the sample thought in these clear-cut terms. One girl, for example, said:

> 'If someone said to me what nationality are you, I would say I am English. I wouldn't say I'm half Nigerian. But if I have to write it down on a form, I would say I was half Nigerian. I would like to say to the person, like my dad is Nigerian, but I would still consider myself English. [*So why would you write half Nigerian on a form?*] I don't know, writing it down is sort of stating exactly what you are. I'm half Nigerian, half English.'

However, a large majority of the mixed-parentage sample thought of themselves as either English (in 50 per cent of cases) or British (in 24 per cent of cases). For the rest, one boy described himself as a European, and two girls were uncertain about their national identity.

Because we were aware that many white people do not think of black people as English, we asked the young people what they regarded as the difference between being English and British. The majority of the sample defined the difference in geographical terms. But when we went on to ask whether they thought to be English you had to be white, about half (55 per cent) answered, sometimes reluctantly, that they felt this was the case, including some who had just described themselves as English.

> 'I think of myself as English, actually. England is where I was born, and my father's English, and I feel English. [*What sort of people do you think of as being English?*] I suppose I would think white people more. I suppose that's a contradiction, but I do consider myself English and black. The thing is, I do like this country, so that's why I consider myself English, 'cos I'd like to live here.'

Others, however, insisted that English people no longer had to be white.

'Well, I think gone are the days when you thought of the English as upper crust, the English lord. I think London is becoming more and more cosmopolitan, and I would consider myself just as English as say a white person. [I know that you think of yourself as English, but do you think of English people as white when you first think of them?] The very first thing I think of as English, is, I don't know, white men in bowler hats, and Guards, even though now England is such a multiracial coloured place, there's all colours, it's not just white people.'

Those who described themselves as British usually felt that only white people could be English.

'Well, English, I only think of white people, I don't think you'd ever call a black person English, you'd be British.'

'I think of myself as British, not English. [*Why is that?*] I just associate English with tennis and cucumber sandwiches, and garden parties, and things like that . . . British is much more mixed. England, I think of kings and queens. [*So do you think of English people as being white?*] Yes, I guess I do, in a way, maybe that's why I don't think I'm English.'

Even though three-quarters of the young people of mixed parentage thought of themselves as English or British, few had strong feelings of loyalty to Britain. We explored this issue through a series of questions. The largest number of positive responses was in response to the question 'Do you feel that Britain is your country?' Sixty per cent said they did, a further 14 per cent reluctantly agreed ('In a way', 'I suppose so') while 25 per cent said they did not. But even those who said they did feel Britain was their country often tended to give rather unenthusiastic replies.

'Yes, well, now I think about it, Britain is my country, in terms of that is where I am from.'

'Well, I feel at home in Britain, 'cos I've lived here as long as I can remember, but I don't feel, you know, really closely attached to it. It's just, you know, somewhere where I've lived all my life.'

One girl, who had been educated in Britain, had parents whose work had taken them to a number of countries.

'I don't feel any country is my country. I think that's just part of being brown, and part of having travelled so much. I say home's everywhere, really. It might mean my aunt's house in London, or where I was born, or where my parents are living now.'

The concept of loyalty probably implies a higher level of commitment than recognising a country as 'mine'; only one-third of the mixed-parentage group said that they felt loyal to Britain. The same proportion said they felt loyal to their black parent's country of origin. Some of these young people felt loyal to both, although not always equally so: 'I do feel loyal to Jamaica, but more loyal to Britain, because that is where I am from.'
Others felt loyalty to one country only.

'I do feel loyal to Britain. Trinidad? Oh, that's a problem, it's so far away, and I've only visited it once, I don't think I would really'.

'Sometimes, when I go abroad, I feel, you know, you have to try and act in a certain way, 'cos you don't want to give Britain a bad name. In that respect, I probably am a bit attached to it. But I don't feel that attached to it because I don't actually think much of the Government and the Royal Family, I'm not always defending it whenever anyone's being nasty about it. [*And Nigeria?*] Yes, I feel loyal to Nigeria. [*Why is that?*] Probably 'cos it's a Third World country, I feel like it's got more to lose than Britain. I think a lot of British people are, like, really arrogant, and I think Nigerian people are still struggling, and they're trying to make the most of it, where a lot of British people don't realise what they've got. Also as I was born there, I feel as if I've got my early roots there as well.' [This girl moved to London when she was 4.]

However, half the sample, 48 per cent, said that they did not feel loyal to any country. Both the concept of loyalty, and an even less popular concept, patriotism, tended to be associated with support for the Government and the Royal Family, and jingoistic attitudes.

'Loyal? Not at the moment, Britain sort of gets on my nerves a bit at the moment, because I don't particularly agree with the Conservative government, so I disagree with whatever Britain does.'

[*Loyal?*] 'No, it's not that I don't really care, but I wouldn't go fighting any wars on behalf of England, apart from things like

World War 2 because of the Nazis. [*Do you feel loyalty to Guyana?*] Only in the sense that it needs it more, it needs more positive attention than England does, but I don't really feel loyal to Guyana.'

Sixty per cent of the young people of mixed parentage said they did not feel patriotic about any country.

'No, 'cos I don't like patriotism, 'cos it leads to all sorts of problems. I mean, it's good to be proud, but the word patriotism's a bit, it sort of causes some problems. [*What do you mean by that?*] Jingoism, xenophobia. . . . You should be proud of your country, but not so that you think you're better than other people because you come from a certain country.'

Only 20 per cent felt patriotic to Britain, including 7 per cent who also felt patriotic to their black parent's country of origin.

'I love England, I couldn't live anywhere else, and when people criticise England and English people I feel hurt, that is how I define patriotism.'

[*Would you call yourself patriotic?*] 'Yes, I suppose so. I hate people who are always putting down England, or North American people who say we are quaint, and I feel I have to speak up. I really do like England, I don't think I would like to live anywhere else.'

Only 4 per cent felt patriotic about their black parent's country of origin but not about Britain, while 16 per cent did not understand the term.

Support for national teams in the Olympic games was more widely accepted. Support for British teams (by 33 per cent of the sample) was slightly greater than support for teams from their black parent's country (26 per cent). The rest of the sample said they did not support either country, but had their favourite teams or supported the best teams; three young people said they supported any with black players.

Because the emotional tie to both countries was usually weak, no deep conflict of loyalties was described. One girl, who thought of herself as English, when asked if she supported British teams in the Olympics, answered:

'Yeah, in a way I feel proud, the way we're improving, you know. But I also feel proud when Nigerian people win something.

[*Supposing it were England and Nigeria, which would you support?*] Probably Nigeria, I think. It's only because they're not so good, you know, I don't know, I just feel as if they need more encouragement, more than the British.'

A boy who lived with his Trinidadian mother, and had visited Trinidad when he was 10, said:

'No, I don't support their teams, but I do feel a bit more interested, I look at them in a slightly different way. [*Do you identify with them at all?*] No, I just look at them and think Oh, my mum's from there.'

The strongest identity for many of our sample was as a Londoner. When asked if they felt more of a Londoner than English (or British, or Caribbean) two-thirds of the sample said they did.

'Yes, definitely, there is so much to do, and it is multicultural, you get a variety of different food and things, I find it is really nice because it is so varied.'

'I personally think of English as being posh and things like that, but a Londoner is just a normal common person.'

'Yes, because you know this is where I have been brought up, and I know my way around it well, I know a lot of people, and I feel at ease, you know.'

Religious allegiances

Because of the strong religious beliefs of many Africans and African Caribbeans, we thought it possible that religion might form part of the young people's cultural allegiance. In fact, only 11 per cent of the young people said that religion was an important part of their lives, compared with 28 per cent of the black sample, and 20 per cent of the white sample. None belonged to a specifically black church. The girl for whom religion was most important was, like her white mother, a Jehovah's Witness. Her out-of-school activities and friendships were entirely centred on the church. Some of the young people said their African fathers were Muslim, but they themselves were not. Of those who currently or in the past had some religious affiliation, most had been Roman Catholic, or members of the Church of England.

Perceived boundaries between black and white people and cultures

In order to have a strong sense of oneself as a member of a black or white group one must perceive these two groups as having distinct characteristics and cultures. It was clear that this perception was not shared by all of our sample. One-third of the mixed-parentage sample felt that their past and future lives had not been, and would not be, different if they were either black or white, instead of being of mixed parentage. Two-thirds felt equally comfortable with black and white people, and three-quarters felt that one cannot generalise about the characteristics of black and white people. Only a quarter thought that black and white people have different tastes in music and fashion, with the majority arguing that some did and some did not. Seventy per cent said that their colour had never prevented them from doing something they wanted to do.

We gave each of the young people a score for their perception of the strength of black–white boundaries, based on their responses to the questions listed above. Their scores were not related to background factors such as social class, gender, and the racial mix of their family and school. They were related to the extent of their experience of racism, with those reporting greater experience perceiving stronger boundaries (Table 7.6: see Appendix).

Summary and discussion

The great majority of the sample did not experience the feelings of social isolation and rejection by both black and white groups which the marginality theorists described as 'their fate' (Chapter 3). It is true that most had experienced racism from white people, and some had been discriminated against by black people, but they also had many white and black friends. They were not rejected by their white peers – virtually all had at least one white friend. In fact, their friends, and their close friends, were twice as likely to be white as black. Only a minority (30 per cent) bridged both cultures in the sense of having both black and white close friends, and both black and white boyfriends or girlfriends.

This preponderance of close relationships with white people was related to attending mainly white schools and independent schools. A small minority felt uncomfortable with, and negative about, black people, or afraid of black males, and two or three felt that black people were hostile to them. The great majority said they felt comfortable with both black and white people, that they would prefer to live in a mixed (rather than a black or white) neighbourhood and that they had no colour preference for a marriage partner. It was certainly not the case, as asserted by some social workers, that those young people who lived only with a white parent would be unable to relate to black people. In fact the reverse was the case – those living with a white parent or parents tended to have a stronger affiliation to black people than those living with black parents.

The reason for this seemed to be the tendency in our sample for families with one or two black parents to send their children to predominantly white schools. There was a very significant relationship between the colour mix of the school and affiliation to black or white people, with those attending predominantly white schools, and independent schools, being more affiliated to white people, and those attending multiracial schools, to black people. Often, these black parents lived in predominantly white areas, and some had mainly white friends themselves, so that the young people had virtually no access to black people other than their parents. It is not surprising that a few of the young people had internalised white standards of beauty, and white fears of black males.

In a similar way, it was not the colour mix of the family but the colour mix of the school and also the social class of the family that were related to whether the young people were involved in black youth culture. Young people from working-class families, attending multiracial schools and state schools, were those most likely to admire black music forms, wear black fashions and listen to black radio stations. But many young people implicitly or explicitly resisted the idea that there are separate and distinct black and white cultures. Only a quarter thought that black and white people have different tastes in music and fashion, the majority arguing that there was a good deal of overlap.

Links with African and Caribbean culture, except with respect to tastes in food, seemed tenuous. Two-thirds of the young people (they were significantly more often from working-class families) said they liked African or Caribbean food, two-thirds liked British food, and 40 per cent liked both. Very few read the British Caribbean press. Only one-fifth thought of themselves as half or wholly of the nationality of their black parent: the great majority thought of themselves as English or British. This was in some cases combined with a feeling of loyalty to their black parent's country. The same proportion (one-third) said they felt loyal to England and to their parent's country, while slightly more said they felt patriotic about England rather than about their parent's country, and slightly more supported British rather than African or Caribbean teams. But the emotional charge of their loyalty to either country seemed in most cases to be weak. Half said they did not feel loyal to any country, and more than half said they did not feel patriotic about any country. Over one-third did not expect to live in Britain, but their sights were set on the USA and Europe, not Africa and the Caribbean.

Part of the reason for the lack of warmth in their feeling about England was probably the view, expressed by half of them, that to be English is to be white. For this reason, even for those who thought of themselves as English, their Englishness was problematic. They tended to associate the concept 'English' with kings and queens and the life of the white upper class, in which they had no part. For this reason some preferred 'British' as a more accessible, and hence lower status, identity. 'Londoner' was the most acceptable identity, preferred to any national identity by two-thirds of the sample. Many had a strong emotional tie to London, not because of any historical associations, but precisely because they saw it as a new and burgeoning multiracial society, where they knew their way around, in many senses, and felt relatively secure. The same attitudes were held by a larger proportion of those with two black parents, and even some of the young white people had 'vacated' or abandoned the notion of Englishness as a national identity (see Back, 1996; Phoenix, 1997).

8   Experiencing racism

In this chapter we describe the young people's accounts of their experience of racism. The definition of racism is a controversial issue. Some regard racism as a form of prejudice, based on an individual's ignorance of, and hostility towards, a racial group seen as alien. Others regard it as a societal, rather than an individual, phenomenon. According to this view, racism is a set of social practices which changes over time and across social contexts, and which is used to maintain the status quo with respect to the power relationship between the white majority and other, minority, ethnic groups. While there are common features of racism, it affects different groups of people in different ways, depending, for example, on gender, social class and ethnicity. For this reason it is now often theorised in the plural, as racisms. 'Institutional racism', whereby racism is perpetuated in the ways institutions operate, without the individuals who have power in the institution necessarily holding a racist ideology themselves, is an example of such a practice.

It will be clear in the discussion which follows that all the young people in our study held a variant of the first view of racism. When we asked them early in the interview what they understood by racism, the great majority (79 per cent) said it was racially prejudiced behaviour which anyone can show, while the rest said the behaviour was usually from white to black people. No one said it could only be from white people, or mentioned institutional racism, and the examples they gave of racism included discriminatory behaviour of black people to Asian or white people. Since our aim in this book is to describe the young people's views, we recount their experiences of racism as they saw it.

Racist name-calling: in the past

'Yellow belly', 'half-breed', 'breed' and 'redskin' were the commonest taunts thrown at the mixed-parentage young people. Like those with two black parents, they were also called 'nigger', 'jungle bunny', 'Zulu', 'blacky', 'wog' and 'gollywog'. They were told that they had been in the oven or toaster too long, or that they were an overdone chicken. Those with a black mother might hear her referred to as a 'black bitch', those with a white mother, as a 'black man's fucker'. Contrary to what is often believed, the young people said that these insults were much more common in primary than in secondary school. The mixed-parentage sample had received them just as often as the black children. Seventy-two per cent of the mixed-parentage group said they had been called names in the past, including 22 per cent who said that this had happened often. (The comparable proportions for the black group were 73 per cent and 19 per cent.)

While some white people might consider such insults to be part and parcel of playground life, there is no doubt that a number of the children found them deeply distressing.

'It was when I was 9 or 10, and we moved to X [an outer suburb] and there was no black people up there, and I got called names, blacky, nigger. I couldn't understand it, I mean, I was a person, it's just that the colour of my skin was different. I had friends, white friends, and they were really good to me, but it was these boys, they used to call me names, and it used to upset me. And they didn't like my mum, because my mum lived with a black man. And my parents didn't want me to grow up being upset and hurt, so we moved back to Y' [a racially mixed area].

'In my junior school, which was mostly a white school, I was called things like "wog" and "chocolate face". I mean, they may sound silly, but then it really hurt, especially as you were growing up then, and not fully aware of the situation, and you think, why are they singling me out?, and that can really hurt. I think when you get called names when you're younger, that can affect you for quite a long time, because you keep thinking about it, and you get hurt easier then. Lots of people, if they make a racist remark, they don't really notice it, but the person who has been called it does, and it affects them, I think. [*Did that happen many times?*] No, only a few, it wasn't like every day being pestered, and going home crying, it was just little remarks, like "You don't belong in this country", and then you don't know what you've done. But it's only been a few times, it doesn't happen now. [*Not at all?*] No, not now.'

Name-calling was often the occasion when the children first became aware of their colour.

'I was about 6 or 7, and I was in the park, and there's some black girls, and they starts shouting at me, about being a half-caste. I felt angry, I just didn't play in the park again.'

In other instances they were made unpleasantly aware of their 'difference' by the comments of other children.

'It was in junior school when, like, people used to ask me, "What colour is your dad? What colour is your mum?" That made me realise that it isn't normal, or they think it isn't normal, for someone to have a black dad and a white mum. That made me feel different, and I never used to like it, but now I know it doesn't matter.'

In these two instances, the comments came from black as well as white children. This was the case with 20 per cent of those who reported name-calling, although usually they said more white than black children had been involved.

Some children became aware of their colour when they saw *others* being subjected to discrimination. The girl quoted below was frightened that this discrimination would be extended to her. She tried to prevent this from happening by allying herself with the white children.

'It was in the nursery, the Indian, Pakistani children were bullied, they were left out of things, people would be very angry if a teacher put them as their partner, and if they were in the sandpit or whatever they'd be kicked out. And people didn't get to know them at all. And that carried on at primary school. I tried my best, in the scope of how much my friends would allow me, to be friendly with them. But if it was apparent that I was doing the wrong thing by talking, say, to an Indian child, then I would have gone off and left them. Because I was so worried that it would turn round, and I would be the subject of it, that I wanted to keep as much as I could in favour. I was just very scared that I would be discriminated against. . . . And so I wanted to be white at the time, to fit in, because I was in a very nasty group of people. They were very nasty girls, all white, except me and one other girl, who was Guyanese.

We weren't considered coloured at all, we were considered white, one of them.'

However, in the case of half the sample (55 per cent) their first awareness of colour was not associated with unhappy feelings.

'Oh God, I don't know, probably when I was about 2. [*Was there any particular incident?*] I don't think so, no, I knew when I was quite young that I was half black and half white, and I mean I've always liked being this colour . . . I kind of grew into being aware of colour, and I think I'm realising more about it because of what you hear in the media, what you read in the newspapers.'

'I was in a primary school in X, which is a pretty rough area, there is racism there as well, but at school I never got any racial harassment, maybe they would use words, but they wouldn't actually know what they meant, and we would think nothing of it. It was a very good school, in other schools I'm sure it was worse. [*So you weren't conscious of colour then?*] I was conscious, I suppose I've always been conscious, but it wasn't a big thing, I mean I wasn't made anxious by it.'

This girl was one of the 28 per cent of the mixed-parentage sample who said they had never been called racist names when they were younger. Most of this group (but not the girl quoted above) had attended predominantly white independent coeducational or girls' schools. In contrast, all those who said they *had* received a lot of name-calling in the past had attended boys' independent schools, or local authority primary schools.

Racist name-calling: recent

Many fewer young people of mixed parentage said they had been called racist names recently than in the past (36 per cent compared with 72 per cent in the past) and only 5 per cent said this occurred often. Very few of their accounts of recent name-calling were told with the strength of feeling that accompanied the description of earlier taunts. Some dismissed the recent name-calling as unimportant.

After recounting her distress at racist name-calling when she was a small child, this girl said:

'Since then? I must have been called names I suppose, but I can't remember for the life of me. I can't remember ever being called a name by an adult. If it was something very hurtful I would have remembered it, but I don't.'

Others responded similarly:

'Now and again you get the odd person in the street, but you just take no notice of it. When I was younger they used to call me names like "half-breed" and "zebra crossing", but now it's just the odd person who calls out.'

'I've been called "nigger". Well, I've been told to go back where I've come from, but only really by drunks in the street, and that's just made me laugh, 'cos it's been under funny circumstances.'

A number of boys from all social classes, and some girls from working-class families, dismissed recent name-calling as simply a form of joking and mutual light-hearted insults (see Back (1991a) for a discussion of this behaviour).

'No. Like my friends, black and white, we're always calling each other names, but they're never really serious, whities, blackies, we're only joking.'

'Yes, like if we're cussing each other off, like mucking around. But it's just a little joke, that's how I see it, and that's how they see it as well, but I know if I got upset about it they would stop.'

'It's when I've said things [taunts] to that person, and they've nothing else to say, so they call me something about my colour. [*What sort of things do you say?*] Like if there's a bunch of girls, like Traceys [*What's a Tracey?*] A girl who goes out with a typical Trevor, you know, wears chinos and a tie and brogues, and she wears miniskirts and high heels, and people think, well, she sleeps around, and she does this and that, you know, so me and my friends were on the Tube and we were larking about with these two girls, and my friend goes, "Oh, you're a bunch of Traceys", and she goes, "Well, you're a half-breed this".'

In some instances, especially in boys' independent schools where there were few other black young people, name-calling seemed to approximate more to bullying than to the mutual play described above.

Nevertheless, interpreting it as joking was a widely used coping strategy. One boy at a boys' independent school, who looked Indian, said:

> 'A lot of people call me names all the time, no particular reason, just for identification. [*What sort of names?*] Nig nog, nigger, Paki, that infuriates me a lot, although I just ignore it most of the time, but often I make jokes about niggers, about Pakis, so I can't complain if people call me nigger, whatever. [*Why do you use names if you don't like being called them?*] I suppose you gotta look on the lighter side of it, because if every time somebody calls you it, you got very angry, I think it's just going over the top, 'cos it's only a word, and so I can't see how anybody could get worked up about being called a name. [*So you don't mind it?*] I didn't at first, but as it goes on it gets a bit tiresome, but as it goes on the less people call it to you.'

The contradictions in the above account were also apparent in his response to the next question, 'Has anybody been racist to you in other ways?'

> 'Often, jokingly. There's one friend I have who tries to make more of a joke of it, but it doesn't really come out as a joke. Like, if we're told to clean the floor, and I start on it, I might ask, come on, come and clean up, he says, we're not gonna clean up 'cos you're black, and you have to clean up, and then I just ignore it and clean up. 'Cos slaves were blacks, I'm considered as a slave. It's said as a joke, although sometimes I don't see it as a joke, it gets, it's just very tiresome.'

Another boy at a boys' independent school had a similar problem.

> 'Yes, I've been called names, and just sort of taking the mickey out stereotypically, like doing Afro-Caribbean accents, and things like that. Last year was the worst, it was just the sort of people that were in my class at the time. But I mean, I didn't take offence, I think they were only joking, I don't know why they thought it was a joke, on occasions it's funny, but sometimes you just had enough. [*And what would happen when you'd had enough?*] Well, I'd just get a bit upset, that's all. But I mean it wasn't a constant chanting or pursuing of names, it was just the odd comment, but it was done quite often enough.'

When we asked, 'Do you think that name-calling is always racist, or do you feel it's a bit different?' the great majority of the mixed-parentage sample (70 per cent) thought that it was always racist, one person thought it was obnoxious rather then racist, and the rest thought that it depended on the circumstances – for example, the intention and age of the speaker. Despite their attempts to dismiss their own experience of name-calling as joking, both the two boys quoted above said, in response to this more impersonal question, that they thought name-calling was always racist.

With some exceptions, including those quoted above, recent name-calling was much more often described as happening in the street, or in some unfamiliar setting, such as a seaside camp site, rather than at school. Once past the primary stage, school seemed to be a relatively safe haven from racism for the majority of the sample, especially the girls.

> 'To be perfectly honest, when I'm at school my colour is never on my mind, never at all. It's only in the outside world, you know, like when I had a holiday job.'

But even in their encounters with the 'outside world', most (64 per cent) of the mixed-parentage young people said they had not been called names at all in recent years. Twenty per cent said they had never been called names, either recently or in the past. All but one of these young people were girls, half of them (including the one boy) looked white, and most but not all went to girls' or coeducational independent schools.

The boys in our sample were more likely to say they had been called racist names than the girls, both in the past and recently, and for name-calling in the past the difference was statistically significant. Young working-class people were significantly more likely to say they had been called names recently than those from middle-class families (Tables 8.1 and 8.2: see Appendix).

Racism in their current school

We asked the young people whether there was any racism in their current school, even if it had not been directed at themselves, and whether their teachers were ever racist. Such racism would be part of their personal experience of racism. One-third of the young people said there was no racism at all in their school. All were girls, with the exception of one boy who attended a 'progressive' coeducational independent school; most attended girls' schools, which were mainly, but not entirely, independent schools. Racism in their current school was reported much more often by boys than by girls, and by working-class rather than by middle-class young people (Table 8.3: see Appendix).

Only two young people, one girl and one boy, both attending comprehensive schools, said there was a lot of racism in their current school.

> 'It's mainly between the whites and the Asians. The Asians make it more difficult for themselves by staying in a group and not making other friends. [*What about the teachers?*] Well, there was one occasion in the second year when a teacher talked about "a nigger in the woodpile". I just walked out.'

> 'Yes, it's mostly name-calling, writing on walls, that's about it. Like the other day I had an argument in school with a boy, and he was like, "if all the blacks got sent home and all the whites had to stay here, they'd drop you in the middle of the ocean", and all this rubbish. I think it's the school's fault really, for someone to come up and say that to me, as if to say well I'm a piece of dirt on the floor they can talk to in that kind of way. The school or the parents should be educating the children. No matter what colour you are you're still a person inside, and it hurts deep down. [*Does the school do anything about this?*] No. [*Are any of the teachers racist?*] No, I don't think so, but there is one dinner lady, because someone pulled her hair she turned round and looked at me and said "You stupid black cow", and I told the headmistress about it, and she said, "Well I don't want to suspend you for pulling her hair". And I never even pulled her hair. If someone calls you a racist name you are supposed to go to the staff and discuss it with them, and then something can be done about it, but nothing was done about it.'

However, views of the same school often differed. Two other mixed-parentage girls attending the same school as the girl quoted above said there was no racism in the school. Such differences were not uncommon. Presumably whether or not the young people thought there was racism in the school depended on the particular staff and pupils with whom they had come into contact, and their own sensitivity to racism, as well as the ethos of the school. This point will be discussed further later in the chapter.

White people were the single group most often said to instigate racism at school, and Asian people the single group most often said to be the victims, but much more often several groups were said to be involved.

'Mostly, actually, it's whites and blacks against Asian people at this school. I don't know why, but that is definitely more common than any other sort.'

'Some of it's directed at the black students, in another way it goes from Jews to Christians and Christian to Jews, but you know, from all quarters. . . . It's mostly verbal abuse, that has developed into fighting a couple of times, but that's on a very small scale, a couple of fights a year.'

'Racism is mainly at Asians, but there's racism like from Caribbean black people to African black people.'

The racism described as coming from the students almost always took the form of name-calling and racist jokes and insults. Racist fighting in school seemed to be very rare, and was mentioned by only 7 per cent of the sample. Three-quarters of the sample said the teachers were never involved in racism, and no one said that teachers were often racist. The racist incidents involving a teacher described to us most often were instances of unfairly singling out black pupils for blame or punishment, or not caring as much about black as about white pupils.

Other forms of racism

Two-thirds (64 per cent) of the young people said they had experienced forms of racism other than name-calling, ranging from differential treatment and stereotyping, where the racism was probably unconscious, to gross discrimination and insults. Institutional racism was not mentioned. Occasionally teachers were implicated. In the following example, which took place in a predominantly white independent girls' school, the white students joined the attack on the teacher.

'An English teacher we had once, we were doing slaves, and he had this poem he wanted someone to read out, and he chose me twice in a row, and I got to the stage where I got so fed up, and I said "Why?" Then the whole class started to shout this, quite a lot of people were a bit shocked, and the people were shouting out "Racist, racist". I don't know, I just didn't like it. It was quite difficult to deal with if you're the only black person in the class. It was the only time, really.'

One boy complained of being stereotyped.

'Well, minor things, like it's immediately assumed that I'm going to like reggae and rap. Like, you say you're good at athletics, and the immediate assumption is that you're a sprinter. And I am a sprinter, but I'd like to say that first.'

Discrimination in employment was naturally deeply resented.

'Well, I went into this shop, they had a vacancy in the window, and I asked if there was a Saturday job going, and they said it had been filled, but there was still a vacancy card in the shop window. And a friend of mine, she was black, had been in there before and asked, and she didn't get it either, but they were still advertising Saturday jobs.'

One boy believed he had met with discrimination from the police.

'I'd never actually experienced anything where I've actually sat down and said, Hey, that's racist, until this summer. I was walking home one day carrying my athletics bag, having done some train-ing, and I was tying up my shoe-lace on someone's front wall, and a police van passed, and I looked up at it. Then the police van came round and stopped, and the policeman asked to look in my bag, 'cos he said "There's been a number of burglaries in the area, and we saw you carrying a bag, looking up at the police van, was there any particular reason?" In the end, once he realised who I was and there was nothing but my spikes in the bag it was fine. But I began to wonder whether if a white person had done that, whether he'd have been stopped, I didn't feel very pleased.'

Others uneasily suspected, but could not be sure, that unpleasant experiences were racially motivated.

'You can't always pinpoint things, you don't always know if the reason someone is not interested in you, isn't talking to you, is because of the colour, or because of any other factor.'

'Oh, I don't know. I can go into a situation and think like say, going for a job and not getting it, and thinking, wondering if it was because of my colour.'

Some young people complained of racism from black people. One girl, who was olive-skinned, when asked about her experience of racism, said:

'Once I was out, and some [black] boys came up, and they started being unpleasant, and then they said "Oh you won't talk to us 'cos you don't go out with black people, do you" and I said "What?" and they said "Where are you from?" and I said "My mum's English and my dad's Trinidadian" and they said "Oh sister, sister, yeah we talk to you now" and they started being nice, and I couldn't believe it. First they were sort of being "Have you got any money?" and then as soon as they found out I had a West Indian father they would be my friends. I thought, God, how can you not like someone, and then as soon as you find they've got some sort of relation to you in their colour, then you'll be friends. That's stupid . . . it's quite bad.'

The girl quoted below, who went out with black boys, felt that she met racism from black girls.

'A lot of black girls are jealous of me, because, well, people say I've got good looks and nice hair and stuff, and they just give you such bad looks that you daren't look at them in case they come up to you and ask for a fight. [*Is this at school?*] This is in my school, in the street, anywhere I go, I get these really bitchy girls, and they'll just do anything to have a fight with you because they're jealous.'

Much the commonest form of racism described, apart from name-calling, was discrimination in shops. Nearly half (47 per cent) of the mixed-parentage group were sure that they had met discrimination in shops, including 9 per cent who said this often happened.

'Sometimes they look at you and they automatically seem to think oh, she is a half-caste or a coloured person, and you have to watch them, and you feel that they are watching you, they seem to think you are going to steal something, that does happen to me, but it's not like an every week thing, it's only occasionally.'

'If I was to go into a shop with a load of black girls they would be watched more than if I went into a shop with a load of white girls. Although the security guard, if he's black himself, he would still watch us more than what it would be with white girls.'

It might be thought that some of these young people were mis-interpreting the anxiety which many shopkeepers feel about young customers, whatever their colour, especially when they arrive in a group.

But in fact, although a number of the white sample complained of being discriminated against in shops because of their age, many fewer did so (25 per cent), compared with 47 per cent of the mixed-parentage sample and 61 per cent of the black sample who complained of racist discrimination.

The most wounding form of racism was probably insults directed at their mothers.

> 'They say things like "Oh, how can your mum marry a black man?" Something that happened in the second year, some bloke goes to me, "How can a black guy go with a white woman for so long? Usually they just sort of do it and run" and I got really mad.'

As another way of exploring the influence of racism on their lives, we asked the young people whether they had ever *not* done something because of their colour. The great majority (70 per cent) said this had not happened. The 18 per cent who had been deterred by their colour generally said that they avoided situations where they had previously experienced racism, for example, in the houses of some of their relatives, or where they might expect to encounter it, like the boy quoted below, who looked Indian.

> 'I'm a bit more cautious, because you have to realise, I mean, it's all very well saying I'm proud of my colour, I'm gonna stick up for it and fight for it, but you've gotta realise you can't fight every battle, and some things are better left as they are. . . . So if you see a great mob you don't go walking up to them, and say hello. Some places you don't go because you know about this. Because I can be mistaken as being Asian, that's doubly – because I think at the moment there is a lot more feeling against Asians than Afro-Caribbeans, so that's something to watch out for, really . . . but, I mean the places I go to I don't really have to worry that much, it's just, you see trouble brewing, you look out.'

Another 9 per cent said that sometimes they worried about doing something because of their colour, but nonetheless they did it, like the two girls quoted below.

> 'Yes, once or twice I've really thought about whether I ought to do it. Like I went on a musical week last summer, and I was really worried about racism, because in the country racism is a lot worse, I've found, they stare at you and are horrible to you. But in the end

it was OK, it turned out that nobody really cared, that was lucky, but there have been a couple of times when I have worried a lot. But I have never actually not done something, because I've been determined that it isn't going to put me off.'

'I'm always aware if I join a dancing group, or something like that, I'm always aware if there are any black people around, but I mean I won't not go if there aren't, because that's just chickening out.'

Only 15 per cent of the young people reported having experienced *no* form of racism, whether name-calling in the past or recently, discrimination in shops, or other forms of racism. They were all girls, most attended independent schools, and most looked white. Another 26 per cent of the sample said they had experienced no racism apart from name-calling in primary school. Most of this group were wary, and some were anxious about the possibility of meeting discrimination, which they felt that up until now they had been protected from.

'I haven't really encountered racism, I haven't encountered most of the things you mentioned, so I felt a bit inadequate. . . . [The interview] made me see that I live in a very closed environment, with not really much variation among my friends.'

'I'm so lucky, I feel like I've been in cotton wool, you know.'

Observing racism

The great majority of the young people (82 per cent) had observed racism, as well as experienced it, those from working-class families significantly more often than those from middle-class families (Table 8.4: see Appendix). When we asked them to describe an occasion, 51 per cent of the sample described an occasion in which Asian people were the victims, and 42 per cent, black and mixed-parentage people; only 11 per cent described racism being directed at white people. But although racism was most often said to be directed at Asian people, very few young people reported seeing Asian people being racist. Over half of the sample (58 per cent) had observed white people being racist, and 27 per cent, black people. Most of the racism observed had taken the form of verbal abuse; very few of the young people described seeing physical violence or police action which they considered to be racially motivated. The following two accounts were exceptions.

'My friend has an old Jag, and he's doing it up, and we were coming home, and he got stopped by the police, and they asked him where's his insurance and his tax and where he got the money to buy the car. I thought, Oh, I know why they stopped him. [*Was he black?*] Yes.'

'I was walking down X with my cousin and my friend, my cousin's white and my friend's black, and some white woman bumped into my friend, and she started going "Why don't you look where you're going", and my friend said sorry for bumping into her, and then she started "Oh you black people", and this and that, and I started going "Come on, let's go and get the bus". And then she spat at my friend, and it just started into a fight, and my friend was going mad, she just hit out.'

These incidents were unusual; what most of the young people had observed was racist name-calling and teasing.

'In my class there's one Asian girl, and she's very quiet, and when she speaks she's got a very heavy Indian accent, and they'll start to laugh, I find that's a bit racist, really. [*Who is it that laughs?*] Black and white people.'

Some of the young people were concerned about racial taunts from black people of African Caribbean origin to Africans.

'I've got a friend who is African, and a lot of kids, black and white, used to make, sometimes still do, racist remarks to her. That gets me really angry, especially when it's West Indians making racist remarks to Africans as if they are someone completely different, when their roots really come from Africa.'

A few young people were distressed by black prejudice towards white people.

'I think they have a right to be prejudiced against some white people, but not all. I mean, white people are against black people, but now black people are turning round and doing it back to them, because of the way they've been treated in the past. I don't think that's right, but I feel more against some whites, not all, because I know a lot of white people who are really nice. I understand black people in every way, but I just don't think they should get back at white people in that way.'

Being racist oneself

When asked if they had ever been racist themselves, half of the young people (53 per cent) said they had. Most of the examples given involved discrimination directed at Asian people; white people were much less frequently targeted, and there were only occasional instances given of being racist to black people, the Irish and Jews. The great majority of the incidents involved name-calling. Boys in particular tended to stress that there was a large element of joking involved, and their name-calling was not intended to hurt.

> 'I've been jokedly racist, but then sometimes I've said it seriously, but luckily the person took it as a joke, anyway. [*Who have you said it seriously to?*] This kid X, like, all of us was mucking about, and we just kept like slagging each other off and mouthing, and I just said, "Shut up, you smelly Paki", . . . although I'd said it a couple of times before jokedly, that time I said it I meant it, sort of, but that's the only thing ever, I think.'

Girls were more likely to express guilt about the incidents, and to be aware that they themselves had been victims.

> 'Yes, thinking back, I probably was a little racist, which makes me so ashamed, because I used to hate people being racist to me. I never actually thought of it as racism, but I knew it would hurt, because it had always hurt me, that's probably why I did it. [*What sort of thing did you do?*] Like calling kids Paki, and stuff.'

> 'When I was about 6, this boy punched me, and I called him Paki, or something like that. I was really rude to him, I got a smack for it and everything from my mum.'

> 'Well, I used to tell jokes about the Irishman, you know, being stupid and stuff like that, and a few Asian ones as well. I don't really see the point of them, so I don't bother telling them now, and they hurt people, and that is not really a joke is it, they are supposed to make people laugh.'

However, half of the young people indignantly denied they had been, or sometimes that they could be, racist.

> 'No, because there's no one I could be racist to – like I can't be

racist against black people, or white people, because I'm part white and black myself, and I have no cause to be racist against, you know, Asian or Chinese or anything else. I don't see that bringing anybody's colour in is anything to do with an argument, anyway.'

'It doesn't matter what colour you are, it's what you are inside. I mean if you take the top of our skin off, we're all the same, no matter what our colour.'

Racism directed at parents

We asked the young people whether their parents had experienced racism, or been discriminated against because of their colour. This knowledge seemed likely to influence the young people's attitudes but the question was also intended to throw light on parent–child communication. Most, but not all – 70 per cent of the young people – said they had either been told or had overheard talk about such experiences. The rest said either that they had probably occurred, but that they had not been told or heard about the incidents, or that they did not think they had occurred, or that they did not know.

The most frequent form of discrimination the young people knew about was that from white relatives in relation to their parents' mixed marriage.

'Well, my mother's parents never used to like my dad because of his colour, and they thought he was different from everyone else, but now they're good friends, 'cos like they know he's the same and isn't bad, just 'cos he's black.'

Occasionally hostility to the mixed marriage came from black people.

'Yes, once we were at Kings Cross station, and there was a West Indian man and an Indian man at the barrier. They knew my [African] mother, 'cos she took me to school through Kings Cross, and once my dad came, and they said to her, "Oh, you must introduce us to your husband when he comes through", because they thought he would be dark-skinned too, and when they saw he was white they really sort of had a go at us all, it was quite strange. It ended up with the police being called. I think that was the worst incident I've ever been involved in. I was only about 4, so I don't remember much of it, it was really upsetting. I didn't really understand it.

I knew the basis of the argument was racism, but I couldn't understand.'

A wide range of forms of racism were described, including discrimination in housing:

'Yes, my mum said when they were trying to buy a flat in Leicester after they got married people were just slamming the doors in their faces before they even got in.'

And police action:

'Well, my dad has a private number on his car, and like we used to have a Porsche, and we'd be driving, and we'd be stopped about four times, because they'd say he's stolen the car, and what would a black nigger be doing with a flash car like this. And they'd search it, like, "Have you got drugs in there?" and all this.'

And employment:

'My [black] mother has, because I hear her, she has conversations on the phone with her colleagues, and she talks of troubles she has with a nurse senior to her, and she thinks it's because of her colour.'

Racism within the family

Racism can strongly affect a child's life if parents or siblings are racially prejudiced. We therefore asked the young people about their own, their parents', and their brothers' and sisters' attitudes to people of different colour. We ourselves categorised their answers as evidence of slight or marked prejudice, or of none. Thirty-eight per cent gave answers which suggested that one or other of their parents was prejudiced against one or more minority ethnic groups, usually Asian people. Siblings were less often seen to be prejudiced – 20 per cent of those with siblings gave answers which suggested that they were.

In all, their answers suggested that nearly half of the young people (44 per cent) perceived either a parent or a sibling as being racially prejudiced to some degree. Worryingly, 13 per cent of the young people had a black parent or step-parent whom they saw as prejudiced against white people, while 16 per cent had a black or white parent or step-parent whom they saw as prejudiced against African Caribbeans or Africans.

'Her views on whites are confused and quite ugly. She hates the English more than anything.'

'My [white] mother does tend to blame blacks for quite a lot of things, she says a lot of the time they ask for it.'

Of the young people themselves, 18 per cent expressed prejudice against one or other group, most often Asian people. The majority disapproved if their parents were prejudiced:

'My dad, he himself is black, he's a teacher, and he's got this idea that the majority of black people he teaches are the ones who don't work. He's got like, most of his friends are black, the ones that have come from the West Indies, but the young ones that are living here are the ones he doesn't like. He's sort of got an idea that they're the main sort of ones for crime, and stuff. [*What do you think of that?*] It really gets on my nerves. I say "How can you say things like that?" and he says "You're only 15, you don't know anything".'

'Sometimes with Asians – people automatically think of sewage smells – and I remember when we first moved into our house, and we had new next door neighbours, and my mum [white] was saying like "Oh I hope it's not Pakistanis, because they will stink the house out". And I just thought, well that is a bit bad, because she doesn't know them, that is other people's views, she doesn't actually know any Asian people, I don't think, so I thought that was a bit narrow-minded of her, but that is the only incident I can think of.'

We did not specifically ask about grandparents, but it frequently emerged that after initial hostility to the mixed relationship, they became very attached to their grandchildren. There were a very few, probably damaging, exceptions.

'It's obvious that she [her white grandmother] is pretty racist. She was talking about West Indian youths, the way they sleep around getting girls pregnant, stuff like that. And when I was having tea with her she was talking about my three little cousins, I suppose they're quite attractive, very sort of stereotypically English, long blond curly hair and big blue eyes. And she said about my little cousin, "I think he's quite the most attractive child I've ever seen", and my dad gave me this look, and I thought, oh well, you know. [*But at the same time does she get on well with you?*] Well, no, I

think there's always an unspoken – I've never got around to asking
her, like, do you mind that I'm half black. I think she probably does
regret that dad married a black . . . it's not the normal thing to do
in a middle-class family, you know.'

Who had the most experience of racism?

We gave each of the young people a score for their experience of racism,
based on their answers to the questions reported above, and to some
additional questions – whether or not their first awareness of colour
was associated with a racist incident, and whether they had described
one or both of their parents, or a sibling, as racially prejudiced. Even
though they themselves would not have been the victim in a number of
these instances, all would contribute to their experience of racism.

We have already noted that both the boys and the working-class
young people in our sample had encountered significantly more racism
directed at them personally than had the girls and the middle-class
young people. But scores on the wider dimension were not related to
gender, social class, or the colour mix of their school or family. They
were significantly related to the extent of family communication about
racism, and the extent to which they believed their parents had advised
and influenced their attitudes to racism. They were also significantly
related to the centrality of their own colour in their lives, and the extent
to which they held politicised views, and saw black and white people as
having different lives and tastes (Table 8.5: see Appendix).

These points can be illustrated by two girls, one from each end of the
spectrum of scores. They came from backgrounds that in many ways
were very similar. Both lived with an African Caribbean parent and a
white parent, their fathers were both in social class 1 occupations
(upper professional), and both attended girls' independent schools,
where there were virtually no other black or mixed-parentage girls.
Neither had any black friends, or links with black youth culture, and
neither girl had experienced name-calling or discrimination in shops.

However, the black parent of the girl with a high score talked frequently to her about the discrimination she had met in Britain, and the
racism in British society, to the extent that her daughter thought her
attitude to white people was excessively hostile. She also drew her attention to the racism of her white relatives; this girl's first awareness of
her colour was in relation to her relatives' racism towards herself. Her
own politicised views on racism had also been influenced by the views
of her more politicised brother. She was aware of subtle forms of
discrimination at school, by both staff and pupils.

The low-scoring girl, who was very light-skinned, said she had never been strongly conscious of her colour, and did not, indeed, think of herself in terms of colour or race. Her black parent had never told her of any discrimination he had experienced, apart from opposition from the white family to the marriage which soon disappeared. She had never heard her parents discuss colour or racism, and said she herself had not experienced or observed racism in any form. Like the first girl, she had a more politicised brother, but he had not influenced her attitudes.

Awareness of societal racism

We asked the young people whether they thought there was much racism in Britain generally, and went on to ask specifically whether they thought there was racism in employment, housing, the police force and education. Sixty-six per cent of the mixed-parentage sample thought there was a lot of racism in British society, compared with 64 per cent of the black group, and 57 per cent of the white group. The areas in which there was most often said to be a lot of racism were employment (by 46 per cent of the sample) and the police (by 43 per cent): only 14 per cent thought there was a lot of racism in housing or education. One-fifth of the sample spontaneously mentioned that racism was 'everywhere in society', but 30 per cent spontaneously remarked that racism had decreased over the years. Some took much of their knowledge of societal racism from the media: others drew as well on the experience of friends and relatives.

We gave each young person a score for their awareness of societal racism, covering the points mentioned above. A high score for awareness of societal racism was not related to gender, or social class, or the racial composition of school or family. It *was* significantly related to the extent of their affiliation to black people, while those strongly affiliated to white people tended to believe that there was not much racism in society (Table 8.6: see Appendix). It is possible that friendships with a range of black people made the young people more aware of the ramifications of racism in society.

Summary and discussion

The great majority (85 per cent) of the mixed-parentage sample had experienced racism in one form or another, most frequently name-calling in primary school. While this behaviour is often dismissed by adults as normal childish repartee, it is clear from the young people's accounts that they had often found it deeply wounding. At that age they had lacked the intellectual and emotional maturity which later helped them to distance themselves from the hurt to varying degrees (see Chapter 9).

Name-calling was much less often reported during the secondary years, and was more often described as happening in the street than at school. One-third of the young people said there was no racism at all in their school, and only two young people said there was much racism. Racism was most often reported in boys' schools, and least often in predominantly white girls' schools. Asian people were most often seen as the target of racism, from both black and white pupils. A minority of the mixed-parentage sample were taunted by both black and white young people. Outside school, the young people usually described being discriminated against in shops.

Boys more often than girls reported being called names. For once, gender worked to the advantage of girls. Two factors are probably involved in this gender difference. Name-calling among boys often takes place within the context of masculine forms of 'duelling play', such as 'cussing' and 'wind ups' (Back, 1991a, 1996), and the boundary between such practices and hostile interactions is ambiguous and constantly moving. Moreover, while in many girls' and some coeducational schools the climate of opinion held that racism was 'out of order', this seemed to be less often the case in boys' schools. The amount of racism the young people reported experiencing, and observing, was related to their social class as well as their gender, with more working-class than middle-class young people reporting racist experiences. Thus the experience of racism of a working-class boy of mixed parentage was very different from that of a middle-class girl.

As well as their own direct experience, 70 per cent knew about their parents' experiences of meeting discrimination, and over one-third thought that one or other of their parents was racially prejudiced, sometimes against black or white people. Two-thirds of the young people thought that there was a lot of racism in Britain, especially in employment, and by the police.

As well as being related to gender and social class, the extent to which the young people described experiencing racism themselves and being aware of it within their family and their school was related to the amount of communication about 'race' within the family, the extent to which they held politicised views on racism and thought their parents had influenced their views, and to the centrality of 'race' in their thinking. These factors seemed to sensitise them, so that within the same school or neighbourhood one young person, whose family emphasised racism, would be much more aware of racism in all its forms than another who had not been so sensitised. This process of sensitisation was not related to whether or not the young people were living with a black parent. All the young people were, of course, aware if they were called names, but some might dismiss name-calling as joking. Being watched in shops might either not be noticed, or interpreted as discrimination against young people, while failing to get a Saturday job might be put down to inexperience, and so on.

Whether because they were not sensitised to racism, or because they had in fact met with little discrimination, 26 per cent of the mixed-parentage sample said their only personal experience of racism was name-calling in primary school. The middle-class girls in particular, who reported the least experience, had often led a sheltered life. Their schools and friends did not seem to them to be racist, and most had not yet engaged with the world of employment.

9 Dealing with racism

One of the anxieties expressed by opponents of 'transracial adoption' and fostering is that white families will be unable to provide black and mixed-parentage children with the skills and 'survival techniques' they need for coping in a racist society. What these skills and techniques are has been very little discussed, but the question raised is obviously important. In this chapter we discuss the ways in which the mixed-parentage young people in our sample said they dealt with racism, the advice they said their parents had given them and whether they had found it helpful, and the models with which their parents had, perhaps unconsciously, provided them. We also compare the advice and models provided by black and white parents, and describe the support that came from other sources, such as teachers and friends.

From the young people's accounts it was clear that the ways in which they dealt with racism, their 'survival strategies', were no different from the ways in which we all deal with situations perceived as potentially threatening or painful. Psychologists have devised a variety of classifications of these coping responses or strategies, but for the sake of simplicity we have distinguished between four basic types which the young people used. These are as follows:

1   *Mentally defusing* the threat; that is, modifying not the actual situation but the way in which one feels about it, in an attempt to reduce its painful impact. Such strategies include 'not noticing' the threat, diverting one's attention from it, deliberately ignoring it, or reinterpreting its meaning by such methods as degrading its user, treating it as a joke, or reinterpreting it as positive. The 'Black is beautiful' message of the 1970s was an important example of this strategy, as was the parental strategy of telling their children to be proud of their mixed parentage.
2   *Avoiding or escaping* from the threatening situation.

3   *Tackling the situation directly* in order to reduce or remove the threat, whether by verbal or physical attacks, negotiation, using humour to defuse the situation, referring the issue to some authority, combining with others to tackle it, etc.

4   *Taking steps to prevent or reduce* the effects of the threat. There are many variants of this strategy, including combining with others, learning karate for self-defence, etc., but the variant most often used by the young people in our sample was enhancing one's prestige or achievements so that one cannot be considered 'inferior' to white people.

Because the term 'coping' is disliked by many, we have used the phrase 'strategies to deal with racism' instead. A caveat must be entered here. The term 'strategy' suggests a reasoned and thought-out plan. As we shall show, the young people we interviewed did indeed have strategies in this sense, but some of their responses to racist incidents seemed to occur without such awareness, and this seemed to be especially the case when they were younger.

Dealing with racism at an earlier age

According to some young people's accounts, as young children they were unable to deal with racist taunts, and simply cried. A recurrent theme was that they could not understand *why* they were being attacked. This inability to understand, together with their inadequate response strategies, probably contributed largely to the emotional trauma of racist incidents in early childhood.

> 'When I was about 4, at my state school, people used to take the mickey out of me, and, like, make childish, racist remarks. They didn't mean to be horrible to me, but it was hurtful all the same, and it upset me. That was when my mum went up to the school, and I suppose that is one of the reasons I left.'

Others responded by fighting, a variant of strategy 3.

> 'Well, when I was at infant school, because my mum used to work at the junior school in the same building, people found out that she was my mum. One boy turned round and said "Oh, your mum is a black bitch", and that really hurt me, and I just ended up by beating him, and I really got into trouble because they were saying that I started it, but after I had beaten him up I felt a lot better about it.'

Some tried to avoid going to school (strategy 2).

> 'It was in the last year of nursery school. I didn't understand what they meant by calling me names, I didn't want to go to school any more. But my mum said you just have to, don't listen to them.'

Dealing with racism in adolescence

Strategy 1: Mentally defusing the threat – deliberate ignoring

By the age of 15, all the young people in our sample who had experienced racism had strategies for dealing with it, which had been consciously formulated. Deliberate ignoring was a strategy to defuse the pain of racism and avoid physical harm that most of the young people had experienced fairly recently. It requires conscious formulation, and a degree of emotional control and detachment that is beyond the power of most young children.

> 'Because I was so young I didn't really understand why they were calling me names, I think I was just upset more than anything. But now I just take it as like I'm this colour, and that's that. . . . Now and again you get the odd person calling out at you in the street, you just take no notice of it now.'

Ignoring racist incidents was a strategy used on occasion by all the young people, more so by some than by others. One boy in a predominantly white boys' school commented:

> 'I seem to just accept the fact that it [discrimination] is going to happen sometimes, you have just got to learn to try to ignore it.'

The same boy, discussing his teachers, said:

> 'I think that some teachers have been unfair, but it's just something you've got to deal with, really. I can't hope to go up against a teacher and to get anywhere, in this school it just doesn't work. . . . So that's something you gotta accept.'

Ignoring racism was a strategy often used in potentially dangerous situations.

> 'Down our area, it's quite rough and you get beaten up, you can get

your head kicked in. I usually keep quiet and ignore it [racism]. If I was called a racist name in school I would tell the teacher, and something would happen to them.'

Even those who generally preferred to tackle racism directly, decided at times to keep a low profile.

'If I'm sitting on a bus, and hear something racist, for safety I don't say anything, because they could turn around and do anything.'

'If you're walking past someone and they say "Oh you black this", and you're with your friends, you think, Well, I can't ignore that, and you say, "Shut up you, blah", but in some situations you might just go, Well, I'm by myself, I'll ignore that.'

Others felt that some racist incidents were not worth taking up.

'Sometimes you come across people that are just so ignorant you don't know where to start . . . you can't argue with people like that, so I just don't bother.'

Strategy 1: Mentally defusing the threat – reinterpreting abuse

This strategy involves diminishing the hurt of racist abuse by mentally taking the sting out of it. This was done in a variety of ways, for example, by degrading the abuser in one's mind, or by reinterpreting the abuse. These ways of dealing with racism are beyond the intellectual capacity and emotional control of very small children. But one girl was only 8 when she used a very sophisticated form of this strategy.

'When I was about 8, I had an argument with my friend, and then the whole school weren't talking to me, she had that kind of power. And I got called pick and mix, mixed blessings, breed, and they would imitate Africans and you know say "Your dad comes from the jungle". It upset me a lot. [*Who was it who was doing it?*] It was black kids, and one white boy. And I thought, Oh, God, why do they have to say that to me, but when I thought about it, I thought, Well I'm a bit of both, so in a way I'm better than you, I'm black and I'm white, and I can't ever be racist, so I thought of that and I just really took no notice of it.'

Another such strategy is to discount the abuse, on the grounds that the abusers are 'stupid' or 'ignorant'. Referring to her belief that some black people looked at her and took an instant dislike to her, because she was of mixed parentage, one girl said:

> [*And how do you deal with it?*] 'There's not much I can do about it. I just think, I don't like the person myself, I wouldn't want them to be nice to me if they are like that.'

Another girl described how, at the age of 12, after her mother had been insulted, she was able to use this discounting strategy to avoid a fight.

> ''Cos when I get mad, I've straight away got to go and hit them and start a fight. But [after the insult] I just thought, if that's what you think, you're the stupid, you're not grown up properly. So I just left it. [*What did your friends say?*] My friend, she was going "Let's go and hit them", things like that, and I said "No, there's no point, he's just stupid".'

Interpreting abuse as 'just joking' was another variant of this strategy frequently resorted to by boys in predominantly white boys' schools, where racist taunts were sometimes frequent, and allies few or non-existent. Examples of this strategy were given in Chapter 8. Usually the strategy was consciously adopted as the only way in which the boy could deal with the situation.

> 'I think ignoring it, or just laughing, is the best way, 'cos I mean if you retaliate then it tends to go on longer.'

In other settings, including some comprehensive schools where mutual racialised insults were common, the young people insisted that the abuse *was* joking and not intended to be hurtful. As one girl pointed out, to use this strategy requires a considerate degree of maturity.

> 'It comes up [name-calling] but if someone says "Oh, shut up you silly breed", you say "Well, shut up you white or you black". I mean, you just make a joke of it now. But in primary school you couldn't really do that. 'Cos you didn't really understand why they were calling you this.'

Strategy 2: Avoiding and leaving

Some young people mentioned as a strategy avoiding or leaving situations where racism might occur, a form of judicious retreat. (If done as an expression of anger or disgust it would be an example of the next strategy, tackling a situation directly.)

> 'I try to avoid situations like that, if someone is abusive I walk away, so I am not, you know, in that situation.'

> 'I mean, I don't go to places where they don't like the colour of your skin.'

Strategy 3: Tackling the situation directly

Even though they would resort to ignoring racist incidents on occasion, the preferred strategy of some of the young people was to tackle the situation directly. In the past most of them had got into fights. The girl quoted below was an exception in saying that she might still respond to insults by fighting.

> 'She said my sister was not black, but dirty, and my sister hit her . . . I mean, if she ever said that to me I would go up and hit her, even though she is older than me and could hurt me.'

However, 'cussing' and insults seemed by and large to have replaced fighting. Sometimes, as with the boy quoted below, 'cussing' seems to have been a deliberately chosen strategy.

> [*So what do you do if you're called names?*] 'You cuss the person down, and insult him, without having to resort to any racist name-calling, you know. You just insult his mum, or basically make him in front of everyone else appear to be very small and stupid.'

More often, 'cussing' seemed to be driven by an anger that could not be controlled.

> [*So what do you do when you get called names now?*] 'I will cuss them. I will stand up there and argue with them . . . I mean, I wouldn't walk off from it. I know I should, and just say, well, names will never hurt me . . . but when they're telling you that

you're a black this and a black that you can't do it, because you burn up inside.'

'A lot of the time I'm just rude back. I get in trouble for it but I don't mind. [*Who tells you off?*] My mum. But a lot of the time I just ignore it. I walk off. I feel better when I do that. [*So why are you rude back if you feel better walking off?*] Because I've got a temper. When someone says something rude to me out of the blue for no reason at all I'm just rude back, I can't help it.'

Some of the middle-class girls used a feeling of confident superiority to 'put down' racists.

'If I see someone being racist I always go up and have a go at them . . . I just feel completely angry. I put on my best English voice and turn round and tell them to shut up or to stop being pathetic.'

'I did actually have quite an aggressive streak in me which is controlled now, I used to get into fights. I intimidate people now, I make them feel very small. I'm not frightened to say I find them very offensive, whoever it is.'

A boy at an independent school, who complained of being stereotyped as a reggae fan, used a milder degree of assertiveness.

'I'm not pleased about it, but at the same time I'm not going to go wild and hit them. [*Do you feel wild inside?*] Um, a little bit annoyed. I say, "Well, if I like reggae then you'll know that's how I feel, wait for me to say before you decide".'

A girl whose white mother provided her with a model of non-violent confronting said:

'I stick up for myself. If I think anyone is being racist to me I say it to them, I wouldn't like to let them knock me into a corner or anything.'

Nobody took action over *every* incident; quotations in the previous section illustrate the kind of occasions when the young people decided that this strategy would be dangerous or not worthwhile.

Strategy 4: Taking steps to minimise the effects of racism by excelling

A minority of the young people, both boys and girls, saw excellence or advantage in any sphere as an important way of minimising the effects of racism. Excellence in their accounts ranged from educational or sporting prowess to being middle class or having a dominating personality. They all shared a determination not to allow themselves to be looked down on because of their colour, and the realisation that this strategy required extra effort or achievement on their part. One girl argued that a strong personality is needed to deal with racism.

'You have to have a bit more "oomph" in you if you are black – if you are just a nothing, then people are going to be racist to you. . . . You have to project yourself so that you can stand up to them. But as it is, nobody ever dares to come up and say anything to me, because, you know, when I have arguments with people I usually get really angry and start shouting, and I think they think I'm going to hit them. But I've never done that in school, I've never hit anyone. Because you know they think, Oh, black people are so violent, they have got no brains, they come from the jungle, they only hit. So I would never do that.'

The boy quoted earlier, whose main complaint was that people had stereotyped expectations about his interests, said he had never been called names at his independent school. He argued that excellence at school was a protection against racism.

'If someone doesn't know you, perhaps they'd say that [name-calling] but once you're known throughout the school there doesn't seem to be that sort of problem. When people know you're good at work, or good at sport, they're not gonna say that.'

He himself excelled both academically and at sport, and was sure that with hard work he would be successful in one profession or another.

'I'd really like to get to the top and maybe become the best barrister or the best solicitor . . . but if you're a lawyer it's who you know rather than what you know . . . but if like you're the best surgeon, then everyone can see you're the best surgeon . . . and if someone needs a good doctor then it doesn't matter whether you're black or

Asian or whatever, so at the moment I'm more for medicine. . . . But if I was absolutely dead set on preferring law, then I'll put absolutely everything into making sure that I could show I was better.'

Another boy, who intended to go into business like his father, also felt that, both at school and in employment, achievement is a protection against the harshest instances of racist discrimination.

'You find once you've achieved something and you've found you're *someone* in the school, they treat you in a different way. . . . As long as you work hard you're bound to get somewhere, I mean, they can't keep you down. And if you do work hard and get qualifications, then when you leave school people are likely to think, he's got this, he's likely to be more financially secure, we can lend him more money, say.'

The same theme was echoed by a girl, who wanted to be a pilot, and saw gender discrimination as more of a problem than race discrimination.

'Without a good education it will be very hard for me to achieve what I want to do, because I'm a woman, and in some cases because I'm the colour I am. But if I get high exam results then really I am equal to anyone else. . . . Although, because it's changing, in the future it might be easier for me I think just *because* of my colour and because I'm a woman. Well, it's changing slowly, hopefully by the time I train it will have changed quite a bit.'

Most of those who attended independent schools thought that this gave them a definite advantage. Some clearly thought themselves as superior to less well-educated, working-class people. The girl quoted below felt that not only her better education but also her middle-class speech style gave her an advantage in confronting racism.

'You know, people will be surprised when you open your mouth and you speak the Queen's English, it comes from going to a school like this. I do think it's important, because then at least you're on an equal footing with everyone else. . . . And if I hadn't been to a private school I wouldn't really know how far you can go with your life. 'Cos when you're at a private school it's What do you want to do? – a doctor, a lawyer, whatever. Whereas I talk to my friends out of school, and it's just, take a B.Tec, and, you know, be a nothing. They're not going to get promotion because they haven't got the qualifications. So I think going to a private school, you know, makes you think bigger. And much more, sort of, what you can achieve if you work hard enough. Whereas state schools, bad state schools, anyway, they just get totally the wrong attitude, they just drop out.'

The pressure to excel felt by these young people must have laid an additional stress on them, but the girl quoted above argued that it also strengthened them.

'You have got to work that much harder, 'cos if you get the same grades as someone else and they are white, the white person will get the job. You have just always got that bit more pressure on you. So I always think that black people in general – this is a sweeping generalisation – that they are stronger.'

Combining different strategies

Most of the young people used a variety of strategies, depending on the situation. The boy quoted in Chapter 8 who was prepared to regard cleaning the floor for a white boy and being called a slave as a joke was also prepared to confront boys whom he considered 'lower' (by which he seemed to mean of lower status, more unpopular) than himself.

'If there is someone who personality-wise is very much lower than I am, if they are very stupid, and if they call me something, I find it more offensive than somebody who a lot more people respond to. I suppose because if I have a go at someone who is of lower personality, I offend less people.'

Sometimes a series of strategies would be used in one incident. For example, the girl quoted earlier who decided at the age of 12 to ignore insults to her mother because the insulter had 'not grown up properly' followed this up with a non-aggressive confrontation.

'And afterwards I just calmed down and I walked over to him and I said, "Why did you say it?", and he goes, "I didn't mean it wickedly, honestly I didn't". And I just left it at that. And afterwards I just carried on talking to him as usual.'

To have a wide range of strategies seemed to help the young people feel that they had some control. Those young people limited to ignoring and avoiding strategies appeared at times to feel helpless.

> 'If I get called a name, I just ignore them, but – I don't really know how to handle the situation, you know. Because before if I was called a name, I used to wallop the person, I used to get in there and try and beat them up. And it never did any good, because I would just get myself into trouble. Ever since I can remember, I was always the one who got into trouble. Recently I went to this party, it was really awful, I was the only one there not white . . . [I was called names] and I was really pissed off, and I really hated them, and you know, things like that, I can't handle them. So I just sat there fuming, and got my uncle to take me home.'

Advice from parents

The plight of young people such as the girl just quoted above was compounded by their lack of support. One-third of those who had experienced some form of racist incident, including name-calling, had never discussed it with their parents or anyone else. One boy, for example, who tried to treat as jokes frequent racist taunts at school, lived alone with his white mother, but sometimes saw his father. When asked if he had discussed the incidents with his parents, he commented:

> 'I don't really talk to my father that much, I mean, I don't really tell him a lot. [*And your mother?*] Well, I tell her more, I talk to her a lot more than I do my father. But I don't even talk to her that much. We see a lot of each other so I mean we don't really talk that much, do you know what I mean?'

A second boy in a similar situation at school, who lived alone with his black mother, and did not see his father, answered the same question:

> 'No. She's never seen anyone being racist to me, she must know it happens, 'cos it happens to almost everybody, so I guess she's worried about it, but we haven't discussed it.'

These two young people had both at some time received general advice from their parents to ignore racist taunts. This was much the most frequent advice offered by parents, although only 57 per cent of the mixed-parentage sample said their parents had given them *any* advice on dealing with name-calling and other incidents. (Rather more of the black sample (69 per cent) had been given such advice.) Of the mothers who had offered advice, all, except for two black mothers who had told their children to hit out, recommended ignoring or avoiding racist incidents. The only form of tackling the situation directly, they recommended, was, if it occurred at school, to report it to a teacher.

> [She says] 'Ignore it. If it's at school, then tell someone, but if it's on the street ignore it, because they obviously don't knew any better, and you can't, by giving them a thump, that's not going to change the way they think, it's just going to reinforce it.'

Generally, their children agreed with this advice, even if they found it hard to follow. The girl quoted below much admired her white single mother, and was ready to take her advice on most subjects.

> 'She goes "Ignore it, rise above it, don't let it get to you, because if it does you'll just continue your life letting everything get on top of you, and not being able to lead your life the way you want". [*And do you find the advice useful?*] Yes, very useful. . . . Sometimes I turn round to my mum and say "You don't know about this", but she does, because she's been in the world longer than I have.'

A few of the mothers had suggested the strategy of reinterpreting the abuse.

> ''Cos what I get a lot of is black girls sitting there staring at me and calling me names, on buses it happens a lot, when I go home. I just look at them, and say "What are you staring at?" you know. So I told my mum this girl was staring at me, really staring, and my mum goes, "Well, how do you know the girl wasn't staring at you because you're so lovely, she's never seen a girl like that before". So I say to her, "Mum, be real", and she goes, "No, you don't know what people are thinking". So I've cooled down a bit now, I don't snap back and say "What are you staring at?" I just leave it.'

This girl's father echoed the advice.

> 'Like we went to Jamaica last year, and a lot of people were staring at us, and my sister turned round and said "If you don't

stop staring at me I will give you a smack in the mouth". And my dad goes, "They are surprised, they have never seen a family like us", so my dad goes, "Let them fatten their eyes". It really irritated me, especially when the boys were staring as well, and then when they came over and talked they were so friendly, and I said to myself, I wish I hadn't been so wicked, 'cos I was looking at them and thinking, "Tramps, stop staring".'

Although ignoring was the strategy most often recommended not only by mothers but also by fathers, most of whom were black, some fathers recommended verbal or physical attack. Children were thus sometimes offered conflicting advice by their parents. They were usually scornful of advice to fight, on the grounds that it did no good.

'He says "Spit on them". I never do, of course, it's stupid.'

'My dad's advice, I don't want to know about it, is to go up and box them on the head.'

'In the primary school my dad always said, "Stick up for yourself", and my mum always said, "Just sort of ignore them". It was really tough deciding which advice to take, but most of the time I took to ignoring them, because most of the time there was too many to take on, anyway.'

'They've got conflicting views, my mum says ignore it. My dad says, shout at them. [*Which do you follow?*] It depends what mood I'm in. And it depends who the person is.'

A few parents recommended either ignoring or tackling the situation non-aggressively, depending on the context.

'My parents say to me "Ignore it, if it's name-calling or direct discrimination, people like that aren't worth dealing with". But if it's subtle, try and really confront someone, but not to get heated, and definitely not to fight physically, which I totally agree with. I've never thought fighting was a way to calm people down and turn them to your way of thinking.'

More indirect strategies recommended by a minority of parents included getting a good education, being proud of their colour and, in the case of two fathers, not trusting white people.

'My dad told me not to trust white people because it will hurt me even worse when I find out that they're racist against me in the end.'

Of those young people who were offered advice, 60 per cent said they found it useful, 33 per cent found it useful sometimes, or that the advice of one parent but not the other was useful, and only three young people said it was not useful. However, two-fifths of the young people (43 per cent) had not been offered advice. Some of them felt that advice was unnecessary.

'No. I suppose really because I've always had quite a short temper, they sort of suppose that I will always be able to look after myself. They've never really needed to tell me anything.'

In other instances advice would have been welcomed but was not given. One girl, who lived with her African mother, said that she had not encountered racism since she was 4, and felt she would not know how to deal with it.

'I don't suppose they have [given advice] really. After the incident at school [name-calling in the infant school, when her mother removed her from the school] I suppose if anything like that happened again they would say, tell me, but they haven't sort of prepared me for how to deal with it myself. I suppose if it happens at school I would get into a fight, but if it happened out of school, I don't know, I have no idea, I would probably just ignore it, which is awful, but I think I probably would.'

The parents' own strategies

The young people were clearly influenced not only by the advice their parents gave them, but by what they knew about how their parents dealt with racism. We did not ask a direct question on this point, but in the course of the interview many of the young people gave accounts of their parents' strategies. This was frequently not in accordance with their advice. The almost universal advice of the mothers was to ignore insults, or to avoid or leave threatening situations, no doubt because they were anxious that their children should not get into trouble or be hurt. However, many of the young people knew of, or had observed, occasions when their parents had tackled a racist incident directly. A number of parents had, for example, gone up to primary school to complain about name-calling. Their attempts to tackle a situation were not always seen by their children to be effective, as in the following example.

> 'This was in the past when mum had all of us, and it was like them times when white people didn't go out with black people, and people used to walk past our door and spit on it, and my mum used to walk down the street and they used to spit on us and call my mum a black man's mattress. So she's had her fair share of racism. [*How did you hear about this?*] My mum told me, we were discussing it. She went to the police, but in them days the police didn't want to know about it, they just said, Go home. She went to the social services, they wasn't on her side, they just said "You made your choice to have half-caste kids, you carry on".'

This white mother was still subject to insults of this nature, and was still not seen by her daughter to be dealing with them effectively.

> 'I was at the bus-stop with my mum and my brothers and sisters, and some white people goes, "Look at them, they're messed up children". And my mum turns round, and goes, "What did you say?" And they said, "They're messed up, they don't know what race they are, is it worth bringing children like that into the world", and all this. And my mum was hurt, we were all hurt, but there's nothing you can really do about it when someone says something like that.'

Another girl's white mother was seen by her daughter to tackle street insults very effectively.

> 'When she first moved into the district everybody would look at her and the baby, my sister, and give her dagger looks. She took no notice of them at first, and then after a while she just asked them why they were being racist, and then they started talking, and that was the end of it, so they got out of it after a while. If someone confronted them with it.'

She contrasted this strategy favourably with her black father's strategy of ignoring insults.

> 'I've learnt from my mum to stick up for yourself, not to let them knock you down. [*And how about your father?*] No, I haven't taken

my dad's view at all. His way of dealing with it is just like, keep out of the way. He goes quiet and just lets them carry on, I don't think that's right.'

The girl quoted earlier as accepting her white mother's advice to ignore provocation none the less valued the action her mother took when she and a friend were asked to leave a shop because of suspected shoplifting.

'I got home, and I told my mum, and she was really furious. She rang up the manager of the shop, and spoke to him, and told him about the incident . . . but we're actually banned from the shop.'

Tackling the situation while remaining cool was generally admired.

'My mum deals with racism very well. She'd fight back, but she wouldn't let it get to her.'

'My mum, where she used to work people never used to talk to her all that much, but then she had enough of it and said "Look, OK so I may be black or half-caste or whatever you want to call me, but I am still a human being. If you don't want to treat me as one, then that's fine, but don't ask me to do anything for you", and after that people started talking to her so it wasn't too bad.'

Another girl admired her black father's ability to keep cool with the police.

'What happened was we were driving one night, and stopped by the police for no reason, and you know the policeman was saying "Have you been drinking", and everything, and my dad thought that was racist . . . but he kept his cool and just did what the policeman told him to do, because he knew he hadn't done anything wrong, so he wasn't nervous. Whereas if he had been nervous they might have thought he was up to something. [*Has he experienced much racism in Britain?*] Not really. If he does, he knows how to cope with it.'

There was a marked tendency for the young people to copy the strategies, rather than the advice, of the parent they admired. The girl quoted earlier as saying she would hit anyone who called her names described her mother's violent reaction to insults. (This mother, like most of the others, recommended that her daughter ignore insults.)

> 'I was walking down the street with my mum, and there was this traffic jam, and this white man called out, "You black man's fucker", and my mum went mad, she wanted to go in there and take him out of the car, but she wouldn't take none of us.'

The same girl was prepared to tackle the police to defend her father, whom she felt needed assistance.

> 'My dad got charged with drunken driving, but it wasn't him, someone had nicked his car and crashed it . . . and the police came and knocked on our door, and my dad had to go out, and he was just in a pair of trousers. And I was watching from upstairs, and when they said to him you got to come now, I went downstairs and said, "You can't take him like that, he's got to put some clothes on, and some shoes, he's too cold". And they said all right, and as they took him out they called him a black thingy and all that, and they were dragging him, but I know my dad's never gonna hit them, anyway.'

The boy quoted earlier, whose father advised him that the best strategy for coping with racism was to achieve, had been impressed by the way his father's hard work and determination had led to success in business.

> 'He came over here in the fifties, and didn't have a tremendous education, so everything he's got he's had to work very hard for. At that time it was still a very racist country . . . but my dad is a very persistent person, who if he can't get through one way will go through another, so he ploughed on until he finally succeeded.'

However, he was rather sceptical about whether racism is nowadays such a barrier as it had been in his father's time.

> 'I don't really see that colour is as much of a hindrance in society today as my father does. Maybe I'm wrong, maybe he's wrong, I don't know. I think that's probably due to the education I've had [at an independent school] and the way that I've felt secure, really, in the education.'

One girl had the contrasting models of her white mother's lack of response to insults with the aggressive and not very effective action taken by her white grandmother.

'We went to Hastings, and you know there's not many coloured people there, and we stayed on this camp site, and me and my sisters were getting called niggers and things like that. And my nan's down there, and she's white, and she went out and she went mad at them, she was throwing stones at them and everything. [*And did they go away?*] Yes, but they were staying at the camp site, so they used to just spit at us and everything. . . . [*And your mother?*] My mum's been called a white honkey at work, but that's all, by a black person. My mum is very emotional, she said she got very upset, and she just ignored it. She couldn't say anything back, she's too quiet, my mum.'

Despite these reservations, it was her mother's strategy she tried to imitate.

'She's always just ignored it, or walked away. I just try to act on what she does as well.'

However, a few of the young people rejected their parents' strategies. One boy, whose preferred strategy was to treat taunts as jokes and to ease away conflict, was anxious not to provoke his white mother's aggressive response to racism.

[*So did you tell your mum?*] 'No, I didn't actually, because I knew she would get really angry. My mum would just go down there, 'cos my mum is quite rough, actually. She'd be down there straight away, knocking on the door . . . like if she sees any trouble between two black boys, she'll go in and break it up.'

Communication about race within the family: an indirect strategy

Communicating about race within the family can be seen as an important, if indirect strategy on the part of parents for helping their children deal with racism. In only about half of the families was there any overt communication about race and racism, according to the young people. Of those young people who had experienced a racist incident (all but nine), only 55 per cent had discussed it with their mothers. Even fewer had discussed it with their fathers. The same proportion (55 per cent), said that one or both parents had told them about their own experience of racism. Fifty-five per cent said they had heard their parent or parents discussing colour or racism, while 57 per cent said that their parents had given them advice about dealing with racism.

These proportions seem low, but they are not very different from those found within our sample of young people with two black parents. In their case, rather more parents (69 per cent) were said to have given advice on racism. Almost the same proportion (57 per cent) of those young people who had experienced a racist incident said they had discussed it with their mothers. Fewer (46 per cent) had been told by their parents about their own experience of racism, while rather more (61 per cent) had heard their parents discussing colour or racism.

There are two further indirect, but perhaps important, ways in which parents can help their children to deal with racism. They can tell them that they should be proud of their mixed parentage or proud to be black – 50 per cent had been told this – and they can talk to them about famous black people – 65 per cent of parents had done this. The corresponding proportions for those with two black parents were larger (66 per cent and 75 per cent respectively).

In which families was there more communication about racism?

We gave each of the young people a score for 'communication within the family about race', the sum of their answers to the questions listed in the preceding two paragraphs. Of the two young people who received the highest score, one was an only child in a two-parent middle-class family with a white mother. She said:

> 'I have always been able to turn to my parents if anything has ever gone wrong. Well, most of the time. And I think it's really important that you have a good relationship with your family if you can – if anyone is going to stick around you, they will, if you have that good relationship. I am lucky, because my parents have always been really supportive.'

At junior school, when she got racialised abuse, her parents talked to the teachers about it 'hundreds of times'. They always tried to do whatever they could to make sure people were not racist towards her. When she herself was involved in calling children 'Pakis', she told her parents about it.

'And my mum said to me that I had hated people calling me nigger and half-baked peanut, so why was it OK for me to say it to other people? And if she fought for me to be treated as an equal, how can I treat other people as if they are not equal? And I think after that I really understood. I think it is really important that my mum says things like that to me.'

Her parents had told her about the discrimination they had experienced, and her father, who does Union work, had discussed with her the cases of racialised discrimination he was working on. They had told her she was part of everybody's race, and should be proud of her mixed background.

'My parents have definitely influenced me a lot, politically, and also socially, how to get on with people. When you have trouble with friends they have always helped me out, told me how to get round them.'

The second girl lived with her white mother and several siblings in a working-class single-parent family. Like the first girl, she had discussed her experiences of racism with her mother and found her supportive. And, like the first girl, she and her mother seemed to discuss most issues freely and openly.

'The other day I discussed what I had been called with my mum, and she said did I want her to come up to the school, and I said "No, it's all right, because I can handle it myself".'

Her mother often talked to her about her own brutal experiences of racism, gave her advice, and said that she should feel proud of her mixed background. It was this girl who was quoted in Chapter 6 as saying that her mother had asked her whether she would prefer to have two black or two white parents, or whether she preferred it the way it was.

Five of the young people had a score of 0 for family communication about race. When one, a middle-class girl, was asked whether she had ever discussed with her mother her occasional feeling in shops that she was being watched, or her occasional experience of being called names, she answered:

'There is no point in discussing it, because I know that we share the same feelings. I don't tell her, I just seem to accept the fact that it is going to happen sometime. You have just got to learn to try to ignore it. [*So why don't you tell her?*] I don't see any reason to. I mean, I know she wouldn't get worried, but you just say to yourself, what is the point, what can she do about it anyway. She is not going to go round with you for the whole of your life, so you have got to accept it and try and get on with it, I think.'

The lack of communication was two-way, and perhaps originated with her parents. Her white mother had not talked to her about her own experiences of racism, which her daughter suspected she had, or offered her advice, or discussed her daughter's mixed parentage or colour with her.

The extent of communication about race within the family was not related to social class, or to the racialised mix of the family or the school. It was related to the extent of the young people's experience of racism, and to the extent that they believed their parents had influenced and advised them about race (Table 9.1: see Appendix).

Parental influence on issues of race

It is, of course, possible for parents to influence their children without giving explicit advice, so we asked the young people whether they thought that their parents' views on colour and racism had influenced them in any way. One-fifth (20 per cent) said they had not, 5 per cent said they had reacted against their parents' views, 41 per cent said they had been influenced, while the remaining one-third said they had probably, or partly, been influenced.

Those who said they had been influenced usually referred to the helpful advice they had been given or to their parents' attitudes to racism.

'Well, my dad and my mum are both in favour of black people, you know, going in for top positions, so I'm very much in support of that.'

'Yes, I'm sure I have. My mum, her dad was one of the Jamaicans who came over in the 1950s, and he experienced a lot of racism. He was in the factories, he didn't get promoted the whole time he was there. She feels very angry about that, and it has come on me that I shouldn't just ignore it, if someone says something that is subconsciously racist, or is discriminating or stereotyping without realising it, I will say something. [*That has come from your mum?*] Yes, and my dad as well, but I listen to my mum more than my dad. [*Why is that?*] Just because my dad says all sorts of things, you don't listen to every single thing he says.'

The theme of not listening to their father was echoed by several of the young people, sometimes because they disagreed with his views.

'Yes, well, my dad can be a bit negative, I find him being a little bit racist against white people. I've learned not to be like that, but to try and treat people the same whatever colour they are.'

In other cases, as in the examples above and below, fathers were thought to 'go on' too much about racism.

'I don't really talk to my dad – well, I do talk to him, but I find if I talk about things like that he goes on for ever, so I just say, "Well all right then, I'm going upstairs". By the time I get upstairs to my bedroom I've forgotten all what he was telling me, you know.'

A similar complaint was made about a mother.

'The way mum went on about racism, I felt it wasn't my issue, and because she got all angry I think I've shied away from politics and issues because of that. [*So she actually influenced you the other way?*] Yeah.'

Being given advice, and finding it useful, was, like the extent of family communication about race, not related to social class or the racialised mix of the family and the school. It was related to the extent of the young people's experience of racism, and the extent to which they were affiliated to black people, and not affiliated to white people (Table 9.2: see Appendix).

Advice and support from teachers and a social worker

People other than parents were sometimes an important source of support for the young people in relation to racism. Of those who had experienced a racist incident, the same proportion (just over half) had discussed it with a friend as well as with one or other parent. Parents, however, were more likely than anyone else to give advice about dealing with racism: 57 per cent of the young people had received advice from them, compared with 32 per cent who had received advice from other sources, mainly friends and teachers.

Teachers at primary and comprehensive schools could be very supportive by making it clear that racist abuse or teasing was unacceptable. One girl described the effective intervention of a teacher in her junior school.

> 'My mum told the teacher because it was getting too much [name-calling by one particular boy]. So the teacher actually went to the boy and she told him, if you ever say that again you are out of this school, because we won't have any of that in the school. So up to now he's never called me anything like that again.'

Less firm intervention seemed to be ineffective.

> 'You go up to the teacher and say so and so is calling me names, and they say, "Oh don't worry about it", and then they go over and say "Don't call her names", it didn't usually help.'

Some comprehensive schools, following the Inner London Education Authority policy directive, had very strict anti-racist rules.

> [*Do you think there's much racism in your school?*] 'No. Maybe you get the odd few pupils that call people names, but I think that's as far as it goes. . . . There are rules, actual rules, that say if you swear or if you're racist or sexist in any form to people then you'll get punished quite severely.'

> 'I don't think there is much racism at school, but there is some. Those people who are racist, they are used to the fact that most of the kids are against racism, and the teachers try to combat it as much as they can, and I think that frightens them a little, so they keep their mouths shut.'

> 'This school is really good, they make it known that racism is not acceptable, they take it seriously.'

In Chapter 6 we quoted one girl's account of how watching a play at school had helped her to stop wishing she was white. Another girl, who had not been given any advice by her parents, felt that role playing in drama class at her comprehensive school helped her to deal with racism.

'When we do our drama work we do like racist and sexist roles, and like they have an argument, and it just brings you out, and you can say that to anyone who is being racist to you. Sometimes you can know how they're going to react and other times you don't.'

Another girl had found the indirect support of a teacher important.

'I think my main influence there was my English teacher in my old school, who made me realise that being who you are is more important than what other people think.'

Another girl recounted similar help from her social worker. (We had no information about whether any others of the sample were under the supervision of a social worker.)

'My social worker said to me, Do I feel funny living with my mum, because she's white? Would I prefer to live with my dad, because he's black, and like people class me as black. I goes no. I goes it ain't that my mum's white, I like white people, I like black people, and I love my mum. . . . So then she kept on saying to me, "Well, the best thing for you to do is hold your head high and just say, Well, I'm mixed race, so what." [*Do you think that's useful advice?*] Yes.'

Support from friends

No doubt because the majority of their friends were white, more of the young people had discussed their experiences of racism with white friends than with black. Generally, they found their friends to be very supportive. The following quotations all refer to white friends. One boy at a coeducational independent school commented:

'If anybody was racist to me at school, I mean they wouldn't really, they'd have a hard time. None of my friends would really tolerate any sort of racism. I mean, if some bloke started to hassle me racially they'd help me, they wouldn't just sit there and do nothing.'

A girl at a girls' independent school said:

'My friends are very supportive. [*How are they supportive?*] They're on my side, they say the other people are very stupid.

They're on the side of black people as well as white people, I suppose that's the way they're supportive, because they think that black people are equal.'

The following girl described an incident in which she and her white friends ostracised a racist.

'I've had racism slightly in my old school, and a couple of friends and I just dealt with it ourselves. Well, the whole year in fact dealt with it in a way we felt suitable at the time. Which was to totally ignore her until she realised that maybe she was totally wrong, because she said that all black people should go back to where they came from. And we just ignored her, and after a while she realised that maybe she wasn't quite right, and she wanted to discuss it, which was the best thing.'

Another example of collective action against racism was given in Chapter 7, when a girl at an independent school described how the whole class shouted 'racist' at the teacher. Subsequently she discussed the event with her friends, and was disappointed at her best friend's lack of sympathy.

'I found that four of them who were really more just acquaintances really understood and were outraged, but my best friend thought I was overreacting, she annoyed me, she thought I was making a big fuss.'

In all these instances the young people had the support, not only of their friends, but of public opinion within the classroom. The situation was very different in those boys-only schools where the classroom climate of opinion was tolerant of racist behaviour, and a black or mixed-parentage boy could feel very isolated.

Discussion and summary

All the young people in our sample who had encountered racism had strategies for dealing with it, for the most part deliberately adopted, or at least justified. It could be argued that the small minority (15 per cent) who said they had never experienced any form of racism had used the strategy of denial, a form of the first type of strategy we discussed, mentally defusing the threat. We have no means of knowing whether this was the case, but we pointed out earlier that some young people identified as racist experiences those that others did not consider to be discriminatory.

The question of whether one strategy is 'better' than another cannot be answered in general terms, because so much depends on the individual, the situation and what is meant by 'better'. A strategy may be assessed in terms of whether it prevents or ends the risk of immediate hurt to the individual involved, and also in terms of its consequences, including its effect on the individual's self-esteem, their understanding of the situation, and their ability to deal with subsequent threatening situations. For example, the strategy of treating racist abuse as joking may be a good choice in some circumstances, but, if always accompanied by denial that abuse was intended, the individual may be prevented from understanding their situation. It is advantageous to have a range of strategies. Ignoring and avoiding strategies are essential, since as one mother urged, 'if you always let it get to you, everything will get on top of you'. Even denial may at times offer useful protection. But young people confined to these strategies could feel helpless in some situations. Equally, as many of them had discovered, fighting as a strategy tended to create additional problems. Those young people whose preferred strategies were the achievement of excellence, and actively tackling racist incidents by verbal means, seemed to have the most confidence in their ability to deal with racism. But this could be because strong and confident personalities are required to use these strategies. Young people all differ in their personalities and experience, and some strategies may be very much harder for some to adopt than others.

Given the very real problems the young people faced, it was surprising to find how little help and support they had received. Only 57 per cent said their parents had given them advice about how to deal with racism. Some multiracial comprehensive schools had a clear and sometimes effective antiracist policy, but while their teachers often discussed racism with the students, they rarely appeared to discuss strategies for dealing with it. If any advice was offered, it was on dealing with racism within the school context, and it was invariably to ignore it or to report it to the staff. Most teachers are probably not equipped by training or experience to offer advice on dealing with racism. But facilitating discussion among students (and perhaps role playing) about the range of possible strategies, especially non-violent ways of directly tackling racism, may be very helpful.

Advice even if offered by parents was not always listened to or accepted, especially if the parent–child relationship was not good. The young people appeared to be more influenced by observing or hearing about their parents' own strategies. But in about half the families there was very little communication of any kind about racism initiated either by parent or by child, so that each was unaware of what the other had experienced, and how they responded. And less than half the parents were reported to have used the strategy of teaching their children to be proud of their mixed parentage and their black heritage. While we cannot be sure how this lack of communication affected the young people, it seems likely to have left those in predominantly white schools where racism was part of classroom life, yet where there were few if any other black or mixed-parentage students, feeling very isolated. Those who were able to discuss racist experiences with their parents, and who received a great deal of support from them, seemed more confident of their ability to deal with racism, but this may have been related to their generally closer and more positive relationship with their parents.

We found no evidence that, according to their children, black and white parents gave different advice, used different strategies themselves, or communicated more or less about racism. Black parents were no more likely than white parents to tell the young people they should be proud of their colour. Fathers were more likely than mothers to advocate fighting, although most did not; much the most common parental advice was to ignore racist provocation. The wide range of differences between families in advice and communication about racism was not related to their colour mix or social class. We suspect that it was in part related to their attitudes to racism, an issue we discuss further in Chapter 10. So far as the young people were concerned, those who believed they were advised and influenced by their parents tended to be those who were most affiliated to black, and not to white, people.

10 Some parents' accounts

Even though, as we have shown, friends, teachers and the media often influenced the young people's feelings of identity, they themselves considered that their parents were the strongest influence on them. In this chapter we discuss some parents' accounts of how they came to be involved with a man or woman of a different colour, and the problems, if any, they encountered. We also discuss whether and how they tried to protect or arm their children against racism, their views on their child's racialised and national identities, and whether they had any regrets or reservations about the mixed relationships.

The discussion is based on interviews with sixteen parents, including two couples. All but two of the parents we interviewed were women. Three of the mothers were black, four were working class, and four were single. The majority were white middle-class women married to African Caribbean or African professionals or businessmen, who sent their children to independent schools. All the parents were interviewed in their homes, the black mothers by black women. Most of the interviews lasted between two and three hours.

The sample was thus small and by no means random – the parents who volunteered to be interviewed were mainly middle-class, white women. We have therefore not described our findings in statistical terms, but have rather tried to show the variety of parental attitudes even within this small, largely middle-class sample. Because we promised confidentiality to both parents and children we have not been able to match the accounts of individual parents and children, although we have made some overall comparisons between them.

How the relationship began

When we asked the parents how they came to be involved with someone of another colour, they generally answered that they had simply met and fallen in love: colour had been irrelevant.

'Well, it just happened. We was sitting outside the pub and I took one look at him, and he took one look at me, and we ended going out with one another. That's how it all started.'

'I didn't fall in love with a black man, I fell in love with a man, his colour was totally irrelevant.'

A white man who married a white woman with two mixed-parentage children by a former marriage made the same point.

'The first time I met X I knew she had two children, but I didn't know that they weren't white. It wasn't till the second time when I went home with her and they came into the room we were sitting in, that was the first I knew about it. The children weren't any worry to me at all, it was X who was the attraction, and the children were there, and they were no different to any other little children.'

A number of the parents had already had relationships with people of another colour.

'For some reason I'd always been attracted to black people, I'd had a couple of West African boyfriends before I met X.'

The woman quoted below was an extreme example of this trend, in that at one time she mixed only with black people.

'From the age of 11, I knew I could get on with black people. They were more friendly, they were nice to go out with, I just lost all interest in my white friends, and started going with the black boys and girls. I don't know, I just couldn't get on with my own colour. I think it's because of my Dad. He drummed it into my head that I mustn't mix with black people.'

Despite this preference, she had initially felt uncomfortable going out as a mixed couple.

'I was 15. I felt ashamed to walk down the street with him. I thought all these white people were looking at me with dirty looks. After a while we settled down and started doing things together, going out, to the pub, and places like that. And it was all right after that.'

Some others had felt this discomfort to a lesser extent.

> 'Initially I was very much aware that he was black and I was white, and I think I probably looked for reactions in people around me, so there were times when I felt slightly uncomfortable, for maybe six months. Since then I am occasionally aware of the looks, but it doesn't make me uncomfortable.'

Most, however, denied feeling any discomfort.

> 'It was probably a slightly daring thing to do in the seventies, which I found rather exciting in a way, but it wasn't as daring as all that. I didn't feel uncomfortable, I suppose I sometimes wondered what people were thinking, but not a lot.'

Initial problems experienced by mixed couples

Although most had realised that they might face problems, only one parent said that they had discussed this possibility with their partner. It is possible that they had hesitated to voice fears which might damage a potentially fragile relationship.

> 'Not really, no, we didn't discuss it. I suppose we were arrogant. It was everybody else who were going to have the problems, not us.'

> 'No. We were in love, and that was all that mattered.'

> 'No, we knew that there could be problems, but we didn't really discuss things a lot at the time, I think I was fairly idealistic.'

However, all met problems, to a greater or lesser extent. Almost all said that their white parents or in-laws were initially anxious or hostile about the mixed relationship. The reactions of the black parents, very few of whom lived in Britain, were not mentioned.

> 'They very much brought us up to treat people as individuals, but then when I wanted to marry my husband they were unhappy about it. [*Do you know why?*] Well, I think really because they thought that I would experience difficulties, I think they worried on my behalf, and quite a lot of their friends made it difficult for them. They would never have broken off from me, they will always support me in the end, but they were really unhappy about it.'

'My mother didn't react very positively, but I don't think she would have reacted very positively whoever I was going to marry. She still doesn't get on famously with my wife. I don't have big rows with her, but I don't get on awfully well with her. I only see her about once a year, but I don't think that's necessarily because of my wife.'

But in most cases, the parents became reconciled to the relationship.

'His [white] family were extremely upset, they tried to persuade him not to marry me, but they all came to the wedding, and after we were married they were very warm towards us. I didn't feel any exclusion. We never became bosom buddies, but on that sort of superficial level it was fine. X's mother had a very difficult time. But any woman who got involved with her son would have had problems with her, although I do think there was a large amount of racism involved, an inability to accept the fact that she would have black grandchildren. But I mean, we are good friends.'

'The first time I went out with a black man my mother had hysterics, she was devastated. I remember her clearly saying to me, "Don't give me half-caste grandchildren". So I have to commend her, she's completely changed, she worships them.'

Subsequent problems from the mixed marriage

Six of the fourteen initial relationships had broken down. Two of the women involved had married another black man, and none considered that colour was a factor in the breakdown, although one woman, who had been married to a West African, thought cultural differences had been involved. Indeed, all four of the women we interviewed who had married Africans (but only one who had married an African Caribbean) said that they had problems of varying severity in reconciling their ideas about child-rearing and the role of wives with those of their husbands and in-laws.

'My husband has got very strong ideas about how children should be brought up, it sometimes drives me mad. He has very specific ideas about the careers he wants them to enter, which is a bone of contention between us, because I feel they should make their own choices. Sometimes he makes it plain to me that he wants something done in a particular way, and expects me to carry it out. If I didn't agree with it I would say so, but if I did I would probably do it.'

A woman whose African mother-in-law came for an extended visit, and who disapproved strongly of her childrearing methods, experienced considerable anxiety.

> 'I had this vision, which didn't actually happen, of a battle about whether she was going to take my baby back with her, because I felt that was what she really wanted to do, and I thought my husband might not support me. In fact, looking back, he would have done.'

However, the most serious problem faced by the black women and those white women living in working-class areas was racism. 'Nigger lover' was the commonest epithet thrown at the white women, and both black and white women had experienced other forms of racism, including discrimination in jobs and housing, and even physical attack.

A single white mother bringing up her daughter on a large council estate said:

> 'It was me and X against the world . . . I was once beaten up on Earl's Court station by four skinheads because I was with X. They walked past me and made comments about me fucking black guys, and I shouted back at them, and a few seconds later I was on the floor, and they broke two of my ribs, and X was just left screaming, and all these people were walking past pretending that nothing was happening.'

Another woman, arriving in London with her black husband in the mid-1960s, with no job, money, family support or other contacts, encountered massive racism.

> 'Every landlord or landlady that we went to see made it quite clear that going with a black man made me slightly lower than dog dirt . . . I was shown this absolutely filthy little room in Notting Hill Gate, and I said to the woman, "Do you object to children?" I was pregnant by then, and I said "My husband is black". At that time there were cards in the windows saying "No blacks, no coloureds", so you mentioned it because you had to. And she said, "Well then, you can get rid of it, can't you". There was no legal abortion then, and that was her attitude . . . looking back, the people that helped us were all black men with white wives, or white girls with half-caste babies. They were the only ones who didn't treat us like something the dog had dragged in, who were willing to rent us decent rooms, and be friends, and didn't ask questions like "I've

always wondered what it would be like to go to bed with a black man", to which my standard response was, "Why don't you try it and see".'

This woman said she had also received abuse from black women, as did another working-class mother.

'Black girls, they are very bitchy. If they see you walking down the street with a black man, they think, you know, she shouldn't be with him, we should be with him. They tease you as you walk past them.'

The experience of the white middle-class parents living in white suburbs had been very different. Protected by income, position and education, their mixed marriage had led to irritations rather than problems, apart from their parents' initial hostility.

'The first time I recall it impinging on us that I was white and she was black was in America. Up to then, odd things, you would go into a restaurant and people would stop and look, but it never – it still doesn't really – fuss me. In America what struck us was that we were oddities, being black and white was odd . . . it does annoy me that people make quite a lot of fuss of my wife, and I think they're making a fuss of her because she's black, you know. Say someone at work has met her for the first time, and they say "Oh she's charming". I wonder if I'm getting old and sensitive, but to me the unsaid word is, "Isn't she charming for a black person". I mean, I wouldn't think of saying that to somebody if they were white, "Oh, your wife is really charming".'

'I get irritated when I go to functions, and apropos of nothing they say "Where did you meet?" I find that irritating because it's not a normal question, I don't care a tinker's curse where people meet. I mentioned it to my husband once, and his batteries started up, and next time when people asked he said "In a brothel". That shut them up.'

The white man who had acquired mixed-parentage stepchildren felt that this had not led to any problems:

'Whatever, there are problems when you take on ready-made families and I felt, bearing in mind that where my relatives live they are not used to black, brown, or anything else, I felt there might be a bit of a problem with them, that was my only minor concern, but as far as I'm aware there hasn't been.'

The most serious reservation expressed by a white middle-class woman was that the mixed marriage might have restricted their social life.

'We haven't met any serious problems, no. I think we probably keep ourselves more to ourselves than we would have done otherwise. Possibly for fear of rejection.'

The parents' view of the impact racism would have on their children

Three parents were somewhat sceptical about the extent of racism. One woman felt that the issue had been grossly exaggerated, and that 'it might go away if everybody would stop talking about it'. In line with this, she had never discussed colour or discrimination with her daughter, 'not wanting to introduce a topic that might not exist for her'. These and a number of other parents were uncomfortable with the term 'racism', and preferred to speak of 'prejudice'. This seemed to be because it was a softer term, without the political overtones they detected in racism, although one mother had a more theoretical reason.

'I have always said to X, "It is not that the world is divided into black and white people, that is not the conflict, it is divided into prejudiced and non-prejudiced people, and they can be any colour." '

A white single mother who had received abuse from both black and white people preferred the term 'bigotry'. She considered that 'racism' was used by black youths as an excuse for inadequacy, when if they worked harder they would succeed.

'These kids who say they have got nowhere in life because of racism, have got nowhere because they are lazy. It doesn't matter what colour you are, if you work hard enough, you can get where you should be.'

But whatever term they used, most of the parents thought that there was a lot of racialised discrimination in British society. Some thought that it could be found everywhere, others that it was especially prominent in employment and policing. However, only the black mothers, and the white mothers living in working-class areas, had themselves experienced it. And only one-third of the parents thought that their children had suffered from racism. Many of the middle-class parents expressed surprise that their children had met with so little prejudice.

> 'And you know, it is extraordinary how little has happened to her. All her life I have worried about it and planned how to cope with it when it happens. It has been more present in my mind than hers. In the last few years I worried that when it came to going out with boys she would meet a problem, if not with the boys themselves, with their families. But now I have a feeling that if it happens it's not going to distress her, that she will see it for what it is, the other person's problem, rather than hers.'

This mother thought that if anything her daughter had received positive discrimination, and had been treated as someone special.

> 'You know X is an absolutely lovely girl in every way, but I always thought people told me how lovely she was in extravagant terms, more than they did someone else's child who was equally lovely. There have been times when she has received preferential treatment. I find it irritating, because everyone should be valued purely for themselves and what they have to offer, but I would rather positive than negative discrimination, obviously.'

Another mother made a similar comment:

> 'She has been treated very much as the token black at school, you know, invited to parties, and generally people would make friends with her and with me, and I felt sometimes it was a little bit patronising, but X was a very interesting child, and I think most of it was probably pretty genuine. Being so few black children, I think they tend to make them feel a bit special.'

Nonetheless, almost all the parents were worried that in the future their children would be harmed or disadvantaged by racialised discrimination, even if they believed that so far this had not happened. The only exception was a woman who, while believing that racism was very extensive, felt that it would not impinge on her children because they looked, and were always taken to be, white. The rest of the parents had all developed strategies to moderate or counteract the harm they anticipated.

Strategies to protect their children from racism

Rather than ask a direct question, we assessed parental strategies from their comments throughout the interview. A great variety of strategies were used; the two parents for whom colour was very central used a larger number of different strategies.

Encouraging self-esteem

Almost all the parents stressed the need to encourage confidence and self-esteem. One way in which several of the white parents set about this was to point out to their children how good looking they were.

'She has always said that she is very happy being the colour she is, and I don't know whether that is because I have maybe instilled it into her – I might have gone over the top when she was young, but I tried not to. I just genuinely found her so beautiful, and her skin would sort of glow and I would tell her this . . . she doesn't like her hair, though. She obviously finds hair that sort of moves and flops about attractive, which negro hair will never do.'

One working-class mother used a light-hearted version of this strategy.

'Well, sometimes I say "Black is beautiful", it's not meant intentionally. I mean, she might be in the bathroom, doing her hair, and I say "You are vain, you keep looking in the mirror", and she will say "Well, black is beautiful, isn't it". It just comes out something like that, and we laugh, because it's not something – we don't make no big deal about it, we laugh about it, that's about it.'

Stressing education

A second important strategy used by most of the parents was to give their children as good an education as possible. For the majority of the parents we interviewed, this meant sending their children to independent schools. They believed this would help the children to overcome the prejudice they might meet when they left school.

'I felt that being coloured she was at a slight disadvantage in this society, and going to private school would give her an edge, not the mere fact that she's been to a public school, but because of what it's been able to give her. [*Which is?*] Well, a decent education, standards, values.'

'My husband thought private education would give the children better employment opportunities, and an extra confidence, that would stand them in good stead, because of their colour, and I do agree.'

Hardly any of these parents expressed concern that there were very few black children in the schools they had selected, although, when asked, the majority said they would have liked to see black teachers.

Other strategies

These included playing down colour as an issue, and encouraging their child not to look for racism. Two mothers used very different strategies. They emphasised the need to help their children understand racism, and where possible to tackle it, and also to present them with 'positive black images'. The way in which these mothers – and two others more representative of the rest of the sample – discussed and justified their strategies is illustrated below from their accounts.

Strategies: two black mothers

These women came from rather similar backgrounds. They grew up in the Caribbean, in prominent, well-to-do families, completed their university education overseas, and married comfortably off middle-class white Englishmen. However, their strategies for protecting their children against racism were very different. The first mother, Alice, to whom race was a very central issue, felt pessimistic about the chances of successfully rearing a black child in Britain.

'The society is riddled with racism, the question is how one can enable one's children to develop strategies for coping with this, so that it doesn't really damage them basically. . . . There is a sort of charmed environment in the Caribbean, the absence of overt racism or internalised inferiority. I think that [black] people who are born in this country are psychologically damaged, I don't think they can ever recover, frankly . . . their capacity to see themselves without the stigma of inferiority is extremely small.'

Her major strategies were to give an understanding of racism, to develop self-esteem, and to encourage educational achievement through the use of private schools with high academic standards. To help develop self-esteem, she had told her daughter to 'reject any attempt on the part of the external world to impose a view of inferiority on her'. Further,

> 'I have tried to give her as much support as I can, and to say to her how important she is, and how much I love her, and how much I know she can achieve if she really wants to, and I try to give her an enabling sense of herself.'

Another way in which she tried to build her children's self-esteem was to provide them with positive images of black people, through the use of books, plays, exhibitions, and television programmes, so they would know that 'there are other societies where blacks are not at the bottom of the heap'. However, she thought that this was a difficult task in Britain, because the images were not reinforced by the media.

> 'It is always an imposed view, "Mummy is at it again", you know. ... In the States, the kids get up and see Jesse Jackson on the television, whether you like him or not the point is he is there. There is Martin Luther King Day, and there is a [black] identity that is absorbable in American society, so that it isn't an imposed layer. When I start, I always feel it is an imposed layer that the children have to absorb, so it makes it more difficult for me. I do try, but I'm not sure I get through.'

For her, an important strategy was to give her children an under-standing of racism by pointing out its many manifestations to them. And she hoped that her own consistent stand against any racism she encountered would serve as a model for her children.

> 'Now the minute I stopped reacting like that [confronting every issue] I would know society has got me ... It means that I am in a sense having to deal with racism all the time, and people say, "Why don't you just let up?" but I feel that I can't really afford to.'

She was aware that constantly drawing her children's attention to racism could have a counter-productive effect: 'They don't necessarily accept my views, they think I am just paranoid.' In fact, although there was some truth in this, we saw in our interviews that her children were quick to notice subtle forms of racism, such as unconscious stereotyping, which other young people might not have noticed or identified as racist.

The second black mother, Beryl, adopted very different strategies. She tended to discount or minimise issues of colour and racism in her own life, as well as her children's. She related that a black friend, moving into her road, complained that the neighbours looked at her as though she had fallen out of a coconut tree.

> 'When I went into town, because of what she'd said I started to look. Well, what if they are looking at me as though I'd fallen out of a coconut tree? If you get back into yourself you forget all about it. When I mentioned it to my daughter she said, "Well, if you don't look, you're not going to find it, Mum, more often than not". I'm glad she said more often than not, because you don't always look, it comes to you. But she was quite correct, if you don't look around, you're not going to make yourself unhappy, looking to see who's looking at you. Because if you look at them, they will look at you, anywhere, even in Barbados.'

When her 4-year-old came home from school in tears because he had been called 'Paki',

> 'I just felt like laughing, I mean, Pakistan is so far from anything I could think of, but he was so upset I had to stop laughing and I thought "No, I won't let it go", so I took him to school and asked the teacher what the problem was. . . . Then there's a big apology, and the child comes here, and there are tears from the parents, and dealing with the brat, and I thought, My God, look what you've started. All I'd thought of was a simple upbraiding, but the head got involved, the parents were called up, the parents had to apologise, it was terribly embarrassing. I don't know if it could be described as racism, in a 4-year-old. He wasn't let in on my son's game, and that was the only form of retaliation he had. I was sorry I started it, I should have just said to my son, "Oh shut up, and go to school".'

Although this mother gave a number of examples of racism she had encountered, such as the expectation in shops that she wanted to buy inexpensive goods, it was clear that for her an important strategy was to encourage her children to make little of such incidents. Her positive strategies were to tell them that they must work "that little bit harder" to succeed, and to encourage them to feel good about themselves.

'I have been brought up to feel comfortable with myself, and I haven't got a problem, it's other people who have a problem. I am proud of what I am, and comfortable, and so is my daughter.'

She did not believe in laying great stress on black history or black images, preferring to be 'evenhanded'.

'I want them to form their own opinions, I don't want to influence them unduly. They should be aware of this [black images] but I wouldn't make a big deal of it. I wouldn't say "Isn't it wonderful that a black person did such" – I think we should just take it as normal.'

She was concerned that because of where they lived, and the school they attended, her children were ignorant of black working-class life – 'real black people, their food, their daily life'. She had sent them to a 'progressive' independent school which had pupils from many countries. Although she herself tended 'not to make a big deal' of racist incidents she praised the confrontational policy of the school.

'If a racist incident occurs, the teacher will say "We are only going to have half a lesson, because the other half will go to talking about what has happened". So it is discussed, and it gets quite heated, but it is always kept at a level where it doesn't get nasty.'

Strategies: two white mothers

The first woman, Carol, although coming from a very different background from the black mother, Alice, shared many of her attitudes and strategies. As a single, middle-class mother living on a council estate, she had experienced racism herself, and had been told by her daughter of the racism she had encountered. Colour and racism were very central to her thinking, and she, too, felt it important to tackle racism directly, although not every instance of it.

'You know, sometimes I don't confront it because I can't be bothered. I could spend my life fighting the whole damn time. If I think they're worth it I will, if I can change their attitude, raise their consciousness. But if I don't think I can, I'm not going to waste my energy.'

She, too, saw making her daughter aware of the ramifications of racism as an important strategy, although she thought a balance must be struck if her daughter's confidence was not to be undermined.

'I've spent a large part of X's life making her feel really good and confident about who she is. I have made her very well aware about how racism will work against her and other black people. But I have not every time those sort of things happened [evidence of racism towards X] said people don't like you because . . . that would have undermined her confidence to such an extent, it wouldn't be a very positive thing to do. She's aware of it up to a point, but no, I don't discuss incidents like that with her.'

She laid particular stress on encouraging her daughter to feel that she had the power to tackle racism, rather than just feeling angry and having a chip on her shoulder about it.

'She should feel very proud and positive about her colour, but at the same time acknowledge that because of it she's going to face an awful lot of prejudice, and not allow it to overcome her, but to actually rise above it, not get a chip on her shoulder about it. . . . She's right to get angry about racism, but what she must do is channel her anger in a positive way, she's got to believe she has the power to change things.'

She had black women friends, who acted as 'positive role models' for her daughter. This mother, and the black mother, Alice, were the only two parents we interviewed who emphasised the importance of helping their children to feel proud of being black, and of providing positive black images through books, etc. She was also the only parent interviewed to select for her daughter a multiracial comprehensive school, well known for its multicultural ethos and antiracist stance.

The second white mother, Diana, married to an African Caribbean and living in a prosperous white suburb, had never experienced racism herself, nor seen anyone being racist to her children, although she was aware that her sons had experienced name-calling. It was clear that she did not readily interpret behaviour as racist.

'And I can't be sure that I've seen anybody being racist to my husband, although I've seen them reacting negatively to him sometimes, but nothing overtly racist. These things can always be due to other things apart from colour, unless it is really overt.'

Her strategy was to protect her children by bringing them up in a sheltered middle-class environment and giving them a good education. At the same time, she was uneasy about their future.

'Of course, it is early days yet. So far we have sheltered them to a large extent, living where we do, and using private schools . . . I hate to see the children suffer, and I am afraid they are going to suffer from being black.'

A number of other white parents expressed anxieties of this kind, and none took the 'laid-back' attitude to racism of the second black mother, Beryl. It seems likely that, feeling that she herself had come through the experience of racism without being seriously harmed, she assumed that her children would also manage and did not worry unduly about them. Most of the white parents had no such fund of experience to reassure them. Their lack of experience of coping with racism made some of them uneasy and anxious, as emerges from the following comment made by the second white mother.

'I told them that they mustn't mind [name-calling], that they must be proud of what they are, and happy with themselves, and there are always unkind people who say things that are meant to hurt them, and the more they show they are upset about it, the more people are going to do it to them, and they just have to be confident within themselves. It's easy enough for me to say that because I'm white, and it doesn't happen to me.'

It will be noted that Diana explained racist name-calling to her sons in terms of the moral defects of individuals, whereas Alice and Carol explained that racism was the means by which white groups oppressed black groups.

In company with nearly half of the parents whom we interviewed, Diana said that she had not discussed with her children how to deal with a racist incident. (Those who had, generally told their children to ignore it. However, Alice and Carol advocated tackling incidents whenever feasible.) Diana's reason was as follows:

'I don't feel I should impose my way of dealing with anything on them, they have to work out their own ways. I just try and support them from here, so that they know that at least here they can relax and be themselves.'

She said she had tried to make her children proud of who they were, rather than proud of being black, and she had not made a point of interesting them in black achievements or history. Another white mother, married to an African, explained this view as follows:

'Well, I think it is important to tackle the issue of colour occasionally, but I think if you stress it too much – I don't think it's all that important. In a sense you are what you are, you have your own identity, and obviously colour is part of that identity, but I don't think it is something that really occupies that much of a tremendous importance in a person's whole life.'

Roots in Africa and the Caribbean

All the parents whom we interviewed thought it important for the children to know about their African or Caribbean roots. This was seen as an ethnic identification, and sometimes distinguished from the racialised identification of identifying with black people in general.

'We certainly try to make her feel proud of being Nigerian. Obviously, being Nigerian is being black, but we don't really talk about colour.'

Cooking African or Caribbean food, maintaining contact with black relatives, and visits to their parents' country of origin were seen as the most important way of establishing links. Beryl, the second black mother quoted above, said:

'As economics dictate, we take them back, and I can see them relaxing, whereas you have to be a bit a little bit stand away in England, you don't just talk to anyone you see. They themselves make their own comparison when they are there, you can hear from the way they talk how relaxed they are. [*Why do you think it is important to take them back?*] Because they are of mixed race, and there will come a time when they say "Well, where is the other part of me? This is the English part, or the so-called white part, how come I am what I am?"'

Diana, the second white mother quoted above, said:

'Well, we tend to cook Caribbean dishes, and she knows my husband's relatives, the ones that are around. We have visited Jamaica. We tend to have books by Jamaican authors around. We don't really talk about it overtly, but I certainly wouldn't like to cut her off in any way from an interest in Jamaica. I think it fluctuates during their lives, she is not showing any great interest at the moment. It may come, it may not come, I take it either way.'

One mother, married to an African, would have liked her children to be completely bicultural, but doubted if that was possible.

'I don't speak the language, which is a problem. My husband never has enough time to teach them, and language is the key to a culture, really. When we were in Nigeria in the summer they had lessons, but they will have to spend quite some time there before they can speak it. We eat a certain amount of Nigerian food, and obviously the way my husband behaves, his attitudes, are Nigerian, so this house is half Nigerian. But then on the other hand I am English, and I have the major care of the children. Ideally I would like them to feel totally comfortable in both societies, but I don't know whether they ever can be. I think they are totally comfortable in British society, but I would like them to be equally comfortable in Nigeria.'

However, another white mother said that her African husband discouraged her attempts in this direction.

'There are organisations which help you understand African and Caribbean culture which I'd have liked them to join, but my husband felt he'd rather leave that, he doesn't want it over-emphasised . . . he says, "Let them achieve within this culture, and if they don't feel oppressed by it, be happy with it".'

One mother found her desire to make her children aware of their Jamaican roots thwarted by her husband's uncommunicativeness.

'They haven't got no grandparents out in Jamaica that are alive, my husband doesn't know very much about his family anyway. When you ask him when his mum and dad were born he can't even tell

you, he doesn't even know when they died. He hasn't been back for
thirty-seven years. If I say, "When did they die?" he says "I don't
know, I was only a kid".'

However, her children had a video film of *Roots*. 'They must have
watched it about ten times, they thought it was really good.'

The parents in the few all-white families we interviewed, although
agreeing in principle that their children should know about their
roots, generally relied on books to do this, or felt that they could not
undertake the task.

Parental awareness of a child's experiences and feelings

Half of the parents we interviewed seriously underestimated their
children's experience of racism, as recounted to us. They were most
likely to know about episodes of name-calling in primary school,
although there were a few who did not, and least likely to know
about the young people's recent experiences. One mother suggested
that this was because the young people wanted to protect their
parents.

'If they have [been discriminated against], they have never talked
about it. I don't know, because kids are funny, they tend to protect
their parents from unhappy circumstances. Whatever kind of relationship you have with them. Maybe they love you so much that
they want to protect you.'

While this may form part of the explanation, the parents' own example
of communicating or not seemed to be another factor. In those families
where the parents were unaware of their child's experiences of discrimination, we found that parental as well as child communication on
issues of race and colour tended to be low.

Parents were even more likely to be unaware of, or to underestimate,
their child's past or present wish to be another colour – more than half
did so. Again, they were more likely to know about episodes in early
childhood than recent or current unhappiness. We interviewed the parents of four young people whom we considered to have problematic
identities, because of their anxieties and unhappiness about their colour
(Chapter 6). Three of the parents appeared to be quite unaware of their
problems. One white father (not one of these three), who said he did not
know whether his son had ever wished to be white, suggested that
discussion of such a topic is fruitless.

'I don't know, I have never discussed it with him, really. Where would you go down that route, what is the point of discussing it? He is what he is. Saying he would rather be black or white – I don't know. I hope he doesn't . . . I suppose he is part of a real genuine minority, being mixed race. I would hope that he wouldn't get too hung up about it. He doesn't seem to be.'

The parents who had become aware when their children were younger that they wanted to be white had felt shocked and guilty to a greater or lesser extent. A black mother's matter-of-fact handling of the situation concealed her initial distress.

'When she was little, she was the only child of that colour in her class, and children want to conform, don't they, and she would say "I want to be white". And I would say, "Well, you are not, so you will just have to put up with it, and I am not white, and I have to put up with it, and I'm OK, aren't I?" . . . but for a split second it was a bit of a stab – Why does she want to be different from me? But it only lasted for a split second, then common sense takes over, and I think, Oh well, it is only normal if she is with white kids all the time, and I think, We will work it out.'

The white mothers whom we interviewed and who, as we pointed out earlier, tended to worry a great deal about the effect of racism on their children, reacted more dramatically.

'Well, I think I overreacted a lot, because I had always feared that she would have problems. I don't know that I overreacted to her, but inside myself I would get very upset, worrying what it would mean to her psychologically, and was it – you know, I couldn't really assess the importance of it . . . and I would think, "Oh my God, does it mean that she is not going to be happy with herself?" and "Is it going to be a terrible problem?" and, you know, "Is it going to endure?"'

'I felt confused, slightly ashamed that I obviously wasn't doing something right, and then determined to do something about it. I thought, She's not happy being who she is, and the one thing I must do is make her feel as good as she could possibly feel about being black, about being mixed race. So I sort of totally changed the way I brought her up. [*How did you do that?*] I started taking her to black theatre, started buying books with positive black role models in, spending more time with black friends, all those kinds of things.'

In answer to a slightly different question, 'How do you think that X feels about her colour?' more of the parents (one-third) said their children probably had mixed or uneasy feelings.

'Well, I've asked him what he thinks, and he said it is hard, because he always thinks he is in the middle. Same as my daughter – she's got mixed friends, black and white, and say a girl-friend, black, gets in a fight with one of her white friends, she doesn't know which side to go to.'

'I don't know, really, probably he might feel a bit cheesed off, you know, that he's neither black nor white.'

One white mother, who had strongly encouraged her daughter to think of herself as black rather than mixed, said that her daughter had problems with her identity when she met prejudice from black children.

'It depends on how she's feeling about herself. When she's feeling pretty good about herself, then I think her colour is something that she is very proud of, and very pleased about. Sometimes when she's a bit low, and also sometimes when other black kids give her a hard time because she's mixed race, that becomes a bit confusing for her. [*In what sense?*] In the sense that she has been told from one side you're not white, the other side you're not black, and I think she feels that she is black. People from the outside see her as black, and that's what she wants to be, and she finds it very hard sometimes when black people call her "redskin". She feels that she is a whole black person, and they don't accept her as being one. She certainly doesn't feel white. I feel that sometimes is a bit, a certain conflict for her.'

Another mother felt that her son's 'mixed' identity had been altered as a result of racialised conflict in a multiracial comprehensive school.

'They have got more colour problems in that school than any other I've come across. He thought of himself as white and black, and the black kids would beat him up, because he refused to take sides.

When he got to 13, he decided to be black, because that was the biggest gang.'

However, most of the parents whom we interviewed, including the parents of three of the four young people who had expressed serious anxieties about their colour to us, thought their children were happy with their colour, or at least accepted it.

The parents' view of their children's racialised and national identity

Racialised identity

About half of the parents whom we interviewed regarded their child as both black and of mixed race; some parents, including the four working-class mothers, preferred the terms 'coloured' and 'half-caste'. The rest of the parents thought of their child not as black, but as having a mixed identity, 'half-and-half', 'mixed', 'mixed race' or 'mixed ethnic group'. One white father commented that he perceived his children differently from other mixed-parentage children.

'I wouldn't include them as black, no. But having said that, you know, the chances are that if I saw other mixed-race children I probably would, you tend to think of them more as black than as white. That's because you don't see enough mixed-race children. If we had – you know, a third of the people you met were mixed race, you'd think of them as mixed race.'

None of the parents thought of their child as white. Alice and Carol, the two mothers – one white and one black – for whom issues of colour and racism were very central regarded their children simply as black. They had taught them to be proud of being black, rather than of mixed parentage, and they had not discussed the issue of their mixed parentage with them.

'We don't have discussions in terms of her being mixed race, we discuss her in relation to her being black, because that's how she sees herself.'

For the white mother this could create tensions.

'Sometimes when she's quite angry about racism . . . she starts getting angry with white people in general, and I worry, I hope,

she's not sort of placing me alongside them, because I don't want
to be seen in the same way. [*Do you think she is?*] No, no, I don't,
but I do worry about it a bit.'

But half of the parents had talked to their children about their mixed
parentage, and encouraged them to see being 'mixed' as a positive
inheritance.

'I wanted her to understand why she was brown. And having discovered that it was, you know, part of Daddy, and part of Mummy,
that seemed to be a very nice thing. Because the blackness is her
father, and the white is her mother, and she seemed to love us both.
There are occasions when she prefers the black side of herself, and
then sometimes it might swing, you know, to me. But she had such
an extraordinary father that I think the black side is the winning
side.'

'I think I made it clear [to the children's father] that I would not
have them brought up as either black or white, because that was
unfair on either one. If you bring them up to think they are black,
they lose out on the white side, and vice versa. You can have
the best of both worlds, and I was determined I would give it to
them. . . . They have been brought up to be very proud of what they
are, and proud of their colour, and proud of how lucky they are to
have two countries.'

'We haven't talked in a heavy way [about their mixed parentage].
All three of them have said when they were little, "Why are you
white and Mummy is black?" You explain that they are made out
of a combination of Mummy and Daddy, and that is why they are
the colour they are. It was just treated very matter-of-factly. That
gives them a good sound base, I suppose.'

Sibling appearances

Since siblings with black and white parents sometimes have different
skin colours and hair types, we thought that the way in which their
parents dealt with these differences might throw light on their attitude
to the children's identity. In more than half of the families there
were either no siblings or the siblings were said to be of similar appearance. In some of the remaining families the issue, like many others we
raised, was not discussed. There was a hint that such discussion was

considered potentially divisive, because lighter skins would be seen as superior.

'X has got olive-coloured skin, it is more like Indian skin, and she has Indian type of hair, really, it is straight. Y has proper Afro hair, Z's is long, it is not as Afro as Y's, but it ain't as straight as what X's was. And I think Y is the darkest one of the three. [*Do they talk about this?*] No. [*You have never talked about this?*] No, never. I mean, I think if you talk about them kind of things it will start playing on their minds, so to me I don't think it's an issue to bring up.'

Another mother seemed to think such a discussion would be not only divisive but inappropriate, in as much as she regarded her children as black rather than 'mixed'.

'No. I haven't discussed it. I don't knew to what extent it's going to be an issue to them later on, but I am hoping that they will have enough strength in their own identities so that it is not important to them. . . . In a racist society the closer you are to white, the better you are – that is something that I hope they will be strong enough to reject out of hand.'

In other families where the children's mixed heritage was seen as an advantage, the differences were discussed in a matter-of-fact way.

'X is a little bit lighter than the other two. We talk about it, and we talk about their hair. X's has always been very wiry and very close, Y's has always been a lot thinner and finer, and Z is a mixture of the two. And we talk about, you know, if we had a fourth one, what would the fourth one look like. [*Is the difference in colour and hair an issue?*] I don't think it's a serious issue. You never know, you know, how strongly they feel about it . . . you can't tell with teenagers.'

'They like to compare their arms to see who has got the best tan. But no, that really hasn't been an issue.'

National identity

Most of the parents we interviewed thought of their children as English, as did the children themselves. Those who thought of their children as British did so because of a feeling that English people had to be white. In the case of white parents, this seemed to imply a perhaps unacknowledged distance between themselves and their child.

'I feel English myself. I don't know whether it's being fair haired, that is entirely wrong, because the first Englishmen were dark, it was only the Anglo-Saxon bit. [*And what about X?*] Well, she certainly doesn't seem the epitome of Englishness, because of her colour. So she would have to be British. [*You talked about black Englishmen before?*] I know that blacks who are born in England are English, but because of their ancestry, because they are dark, they don't seem so English as the white Englishman. I know this is their home, and it's been their home for a long time, but I still find it, you know, slightly difficult to see them as English as I am.'

The black mothers whom we interviewed regarded their children as English.

'I think X thinks of herself as English. [*And do you?*] I used to think of English people as being always white. Most of the black people I met then had just arrived from the Caribbean. These people's offspring are now English, and they are saying that they are English, and I recognise them as English, they sound English.'

'After all, they have lived here, they have grown up in a cultural environment that they absorb just because they live here. I think they understand that they are viewed as aliens by society at large . . . but I think they are more English than they are anything.'

Only two parents thought of their child's nationality as mixed.

'Well, by birth of course I think of them as being half-and-half, but by culture I think of them as being British.'

'I think of them as being half English and half Nigerian, but I think they're probably English just from living here. I think my family see them as English children with a Nigerian parent, and my husband's family see them as Nigerian children with an English parent.'

Regrets and second thoughts?

Towards the end of the interview we asked several questions which we thought might elicit any doubts not yet expressed about the mixed relationships: 'Have there been times when you wished that your partner was the same colour as you?'; 'And your children?'; 'How do you feel now about having a child of mixed parentage?' And a slightly less threatening question, 'On the basis of your experience, would you recommend to your own children that they marry people of a particular colour?'

Almost all the parents said they were very happy with their children, and proud of them, and liked their colour, and had never wished they were a different colour: 'I am very proud of them, they are very lovely kids.'

One mother said that she had always wanted to have 'half-caste' children.

'The reason why I've never wanted them to be another colour is that I said I was going to have half-caste children when I was 13. My mum just looked at me as though I was mad. I didn't know then that you had to sleep with a black man to have a half-caste kid, and that's the truth. But [I knew one] she was such a pretty little thing. And I tell my kids, you know, that I always said I was going to have half-caste children, and I suppose they take it that I've done what I said I was going to do.'

However, a few mothers had conflicting feelings. Because of anxieties about racism, they had at times wished their child was a different colour.

'The only time [I wished they were white] was when I was trying to remarry, and I realised I might find it difficult to find a husband who'd be prepared to take on half-caste children. That was the only time, then I thought, well, you know, it's going to be the one test for him. Whether it did affect them I don't know. There was one man I went out with for some time, but I don't think it was their colour that put him off, I think it was just the fact that they were young children, his own had grown up.'

The reservations of some of the mothers centred on their anxiety that their children would suffer from racism, even though the young people had met with very limited racism to date.

'I've only wished it [that she was white] when I have worried that maybe it was going to be a problem for her. [*Was that earlier?*] Well, the worry hasn't entirely gone, although it is very, very much reduced. It is just that every so often over the years I thought there was going to be – I thought now in her teenage years it might suddenly become a problem, then again it doesn't seem to have . . . I worried very much more than was necessary.'

'I wouldn't have them otherwise. I don't know if it is at all unfair on them to have brought them into the world and left them to face problems. I mean, I have always wondered whether it was fair to have children. Initially I thought that if we loved them enough that would compensate for anything else they might experience, but I think that was a very naive view. I have also thought that the more such children exist, the less of a problem it will be, because they won't be so strange, and they won't be stared at so much. I don't know, it happened, I love them, I don't regret it.'

A single mother had met with a good deal of racism, but thought it had all been worth while.

'In the beginning I found out that it wasn't as straightforward as I thought it was going to be, and there were an awful lot of problems. I had a lot of racism directed at me, but it's made me a lot stronger, it's made me aware of things I didn't believe existed . . . and it's absolutely the best thing I've ever done.'

None of the parents expressed reservations about the colour of their partner, although some said they wished the cultural differences between them did not exist. This point emerged more strongly when we asked them whether they would recommend to their children that they marry someone of a particular colour. While slightly over half said they would leave it entirely to them, four women who were – or had been – married to Africans and one African Caribbean married to a white Englishman said they would urge their children to consider the implications of marrying someone from another culture. A single mother who had been married to an African said:

'My big concern is that she marry someone she can be happy with. But marriages where your backgrounds are very similar, your family relationships are similar, have the best chance of surviving, so given the kind of home she was brought up in, that is likely to suggest a white man – but love is strange. You don't necessarily choose someone with the same. . . .'

A Caribbean mother made a similar point.

'I think the pressures are extraordinary if you marry cross-culturally. I think that the possibilities for growth and human development within a cross-cultural marriage are extraordinarily great, but the pressures are so enormous that I just wonder if it is worth the fight.'

A white mother who encouraged her daughter to think of herself as black nonetheless saw advantages in her marrying a white man.

'If she chooses a black partner, it will upset my family dreadfully. After fifteen years they've just about got over the shock. If she has a succession of black children, oof! . . . I'm happy for her as long as she's happy, but it's easy to be simplistic . . . If she has children with someone who is white, her children are going to be fairly pale, and if with someone black, her babies would be quite black, and then it brings into question all the problems that we've been talking about . . . I guess ultimately it would be an awful lot easier for her if she had children with somebody who was white. It just would be. But I'd rather be quite simplistic about it and hope that whatever she does she's going to be happy doing.'

Most of the parents, however, shared the views of this Caribbean mother:

'It doesn't matter to me, that's their life. I have done my bit, I've produced my kids, nobody had a hand in my choice, and I wouldn't have the effrontery to suggest to them what they do.'

Summary and discussion

Our sample was very small, self-selected, and predominantly white and middle class. Compared with the sample as a whole, the parents were very unpoliticised in their views about colour and racism. For example, according to the young people, while half had been told by their parents to be proud of their colour, and two-thirds had been told about famous black people, only two of the eighteen parents we interviewed had used these strategies. It is possible, also, that those parents who agreed to be interviewed felt more self-confident about their parenting than those who did not. However, the patterns of response which emerged from the interviews may suggest leads for future work.

Even within our small sample we found very divergent experiences and attitudes, which in part seemed related to social class. Working-class parents, whether black or white, had many bitter experiences of racism, while the biggest problem of most middle-class single parents or mixed couples was the initial opposition of their parents. However, the parents' strategies for helping their children to deal with racism seemed to have more to do with their attitudes to colour and racism, and with patterns of family communication, than with their own colour and social class. We interviewed only three black mothers, but their strategies, although diverse, were no different from the diverse strategies of the white mothers. A larger sample might have revealed differences, but the interviews with the young people revealed no racialised differences in reported parental strategies (Chapter 9).

Virtually all the parents thought that key strategies were to foster their children's personal confidence and self-esteem, and to provide them with a good education, although they differed in what they meant by this. For some, it meant academic excellence; for others, the self-confidence which they believed would result from a public school education. Only one parent said she had taken into account the presence of other black pupils, and an antiracist policy, when selecting a school; she was one of the only two parents in the sample with politicised views on racism.

In other respects, parental strategies to protect their children against racism differed widely. The differences seemed to be related in large part to their attitudes to colour and racism. The two parents with politicised views about racism thought it important to sensitise their children to the manifestations of racism, and to explain to them how it operates in society. They also aimed to counteract the denigrating effect of racism by providing their children with positive black images. In these families the amount of communication about racism was high, and if anything the parents overestimated the amount of racism their children met. Similar strategies are used by feminists to help their daughters deal with sexism. They want them to understand the way in which negative societal attitudes to women influence their life chances, others' attitudes to them, and their own and others' behaviour. They frequently point out manifestations of sexism, and look for 'role models' of women who have overcome the constraints of sexism.

In other families racism was seen in a less political light, as one of the many undesirable, but human, forms of prejudice, caused by ignorance, personal bigotry, or psychological problems. Because the issue of colour was not central to these parents, they encouraged their children to be proud of themselves rather than of being black, and did not feel the need to provide them with positive black images. Some tended to minimise or discount racist incidents, and in these families there was very little discussion about racialised discrimination, and parents tended to underestimate the amount of racism their children experienced and their anxieties about their colour. In all, more than half the parents did so. Not all parents fitted neatly into these two categories, but the categories represent real differences between the strategies of parents who have politicised views of racism and those who do not.

It is not possible on the basis of our small sample to say that one type of strategy had a better outcome for the young people than the other, although it certainly seems likely that the outcomes are *different*. The first, more 'politicised' strategy is likely to produce children who are more aware of racism, and more likely to tackle it, than the second. The two kinds of strategy are also likely to have different attendant risks. The first strategy runs the risk that the young people will think their parents paranoid, and will perhaps react against their views, or that they will be supersensitive to, and unable to rise above, racist incidents. The risk of the second strategy is that the young people will be left to deal with their anxieties and with racist incidents without support, and perhaps to interpret racist slights as being due to their own personal deficiencies.

Nearly half of the parents regarded the racialised identities of their children as 'mixed'; they tended to stress to them the benefits of a mixed heritage. The rest regarded their children as both black and mixed, or in two cases simply as black. These two parents were the only parents whom we interviewed who accepted, or perhaps even knew about, the argument that people of mixed parentage should be regarded as black. The rest of the sample were very unpoliticised in their approach to racism. The problems arising from an identification as black will be discussed in the next chapter. Almost all the parents believed it was important for their children to be aware of their African or Caribbean roots, although most thought of their children as English.

Virtually all the parents said they were very happy with their children and had no regrets about having children of mixed parentage, although for some their experience had been somewhat clouded by anxieties about racism.

11 But what about the children?

An overview, with some comments

The main aims of the research reported in this book were to explore the racialised identities of young people of mixed black and white parentage. We wanted to see whether they differed, and to throw some light on the reasons for the differences, and what the consequences of having different racialised identities were. We also wanted to describe their experiences of racism, how they dealt with them, and the extent to which their parents influenced their identities and helped them to deal with racism.

In the first part of this book we set these questions within a historical context. For centuries, people of mixed black and white parentage, rather than being seen as the fortunate recipients of two diverse inheritances, have been stigmatised. This is because of deeply ingrained beliefs that human beings are 'by blood' divided into a small number of races, of which the white race is superior. According to these beliefs, people of mixed parentage inherit not only the undesirable qualities of their black parent, but also, arising from their 'mixed blood', a tendency to neurosis. They were further stigmatised because they owed their existence to a sexual relationship which outraged, because it potentially undermined, white society. If, as was usually the case in Britain, their mother was white, it was assumed that her morals were questionable. Although black people's attitudes were usually much more sympathetic, this was not always the case. They often had their own reasons, which differed in different periods, for disapproving of mixed unions.

According to American sociologists in the 1920s and 1930s, the 'marginal' position of mixed-parentage people between two groups, both of which rejected them, inevitably resulted in self-hatred and internal conflict, unless they threw in their lot with the black community and regarded themselves as black. In the USA most probably did so perforce, because black people were for long defined as those with 'one drop of black blood'. We shall never know how the small number of mixed-parentage people in Britain in the past defined themselves, or if they had identity problems. Certainly, the eminent British nineteenth-century people of mixed parentage, living in a very racist white society, seem to have achieved both self-respect and respect from others (see Chapters 2 and 3). Eminent people, however, may well be exceptional.

From about the 1960s people of mixed parentage were urged to assume a black identity, this time by black groups in both the USA and Britain. These groups have argued that a commitment to a black identity by mixed-parentage people is their only safeguard against identity confusion and low self-esteem, as well as being an act of solidarity with black people. Although their arguments have been widely accepted by social scientists and social workers both black and white, it was never clear whether this was the case with mixed-parentage people themselves. However, since the early 1990s, when the first edition of this book was published, people of mixed parentage themselves have increasingly asserted that they want to be seen as 'mixed', rather than as either black or white. There is no entirely agreed nomenclature for people of mixed parentage (see the discussion in Chapter 1). However, there is more agreement than previously that people of mixed parentage do not always wish to be viewed as 'black' – even though they are likely to share experiences of racism with black people.

Part of the reason for the shift in the social construction of people of mixed parentage has been the growth in their numbers, which has led the US and UK governments to include a question on mixed parentage in their twenty-first-century Censuses for the first time. However, an important reason has been the campaigning of people of mixed parentage, and increasing recognition that they have independent viewpoints. The first edition of this book helped to facilitate this recognition. We would argue that the second edition is no less important in that it continues to be highly important for teachers, social workers and government to understand how people of mixed parentage define their racialised identity and what they feel about it.

This issue is of particular relevance to social work decisions about the placement of mixed-parentage children who are 'looked after' by local authorities. It is no longer as readily accepted as it was when the first edition of this book appeared that the most important need for 'looked-after' children of mixed parentage is to acquire a 'positive black identity'. However, there is a great deal of confusion about what constitutes an appropriate placement for children of mixed parentage. In Britain, where 'same-race placements' have become accepted as the ideal, there is evidence that social workers are perplexed about what constitutes a 'same-race placement' and how placement with white families may affect their racialised identities. The findings from our study of young mixed-parentage people, mostly aged 15 to 16 in secondary schools in and around London continue to throw light on these issues. This is particularly the case since some of the young people lived in households with one white and one black parent, a few lived in households with only a black parent(s) and some with only a white parent(s). In both Britain and the USA, where new adoption laws play down the significance of racialisation in placement decisions, such findings are important to understanding and developing good practice.

Since our sample were not 'looked after' by local authorities, the findings also throw light on the identities of children of mixed parentage living in their own homes. In particular, they address questions of:

- Whether or not young people of mixed parentage living with their own parents, or with a single white parent, had a black identity, and if they failed to acquire one, whether they fell prey to serious identity problems.
- The impact of attending ethnically mixed or predominantly white schools on their racialised identities.
- How their friendships were racialised.
- Whether or not they were equally comfortable with black and with white people and whether they saw themselves as 'bridging' black and white cultures.
- Whether the young people reported that racism was talked about in their families and, if so, whether their parents passed on any strategies for dealing with it.
- How gender and social class intersected their racialised identities.
- Whether or not the young people reported that their identities had changed over time.

How did the young people define their racialised identities?

We found that just under half of our mixed-parentage sample thought of people of mixed parentage, including themselves, as black. Even fewer – 30 per cent – of the young people with two black parents, and only 16 per cent of the young white people, regarded people of mixed parentage as black. The rest of the young people of mixed parentage thought of themselves as 'brown', 'mixed' or 'coloured'. None of them said that they always or mainly thought of themselves as white, but 10 per cent said that they sometimes did so, or that they felt 'more white than black'. All but one of these young people looked white. Of those in the mixed-parentage sample who did not think of themselves as black, some seemed not to have heard of the view that they should do so, while others had made a deliberate decision not to, often because to do so seemed to involve a denial of their white parent.

The great majority of the young people, whether or not they considered themselves 'black', also used a special term to describe their mixed parentage. 'Half-caste' was used by half of them, and by two-thirds of the black sample. There were social class differences in this respect – those who used the term 'half-caste' tended to come from working-class families, while 'mixed-race' was used most often by young middle-class people. We found that other terms which were attacked by black people in the 1960s and 1970s, and which are now considered totally unacceptable in many circles, were still in general use. 'Coloured' was used by a substantial minority of the black and mixed-parentage sample, and by a majority of young white people; a few black and mixed-parentage young people used the term 'negroes'.

Some varied their use of terms according to the context, for example, using 'half-caste' with their friends, and 'mixed-race' with adults. Although aware of the new terms, these young people were not aware of the reasons for their introduction, and hence were not committed to their use. The political struggles mounted by black groups in the area of language, which had enormous impact in many quarters, seem not to have reached a substantial proportion of young people today. Only one young person in the mixed-parentage sample was familiar with much of the current discourse about racism.

In discussing the young people's racialised identity we have often chosen to refer to their 'identities' in the plural. This is because their self-definitions were sometimes more complex than appeared at first sight. In answer to a direct question, they all defined themselves as black or mixed or 'more white than black', and it was these answers that we have described above. But in the course of the interview it became clear that some had multiple racialised identities. Some saw themselves as both black and 'half-caste' or mixed race. Others showed a degree of uncertainty about which identity or identities they held. One girl, for example, having said that she considered herself 'black', continued:

> 'In a way I know that I've got the colour of a black person, but then I am a mixed-race person, and I can't hide that so . . .' [She left the comment unfinished].

Some of those who said when asked that they did not think of themselves as black at another point in the interview referred to themselves as black. Others reported that they shifted in their self-definition according to the context, for example, describing themselves as 'black' to their friends, and 'coloured' to their parents. These indications of multiple identities reflect the complexity of their situation and are captured in new theories of identities (discussed in Chapter 1). However, for the purpose of statistical analysis, we used their answers to our direct questions.

Which mixed-parentage young people identified themselves as black?

Defining oneself as 'black' was not associated with living with a black parent, no doubt because some of the black parents had told their children they were 'mixed', while some white parents had taught their children to think of themselves as black. Nor was it associated with attending a racially mixed school, or coming from a particular social class, or being affiliated to black people and cultures. Thus some young people who identified themselves as black because of feelings of solidarity with black people were wary of individual black people, and not attracted to black youth culture.

Defining oneself as 'black' *was* associated with a more politicised set of attitudes towards racism, for example, defining it as discriminatory behaviour by white people towards black people, as opposed to saying that 'anyone can be racist'. In line with this, those who defined themselves as 'black' tended not to use the terms 'half-caste' and 'coloured'.

Did a positive racialised identity depend on thinking of oneself as black?

Although recent theories of identities would eschew the notion of positive identities, much theorising, both past and present, suggests that only those young people who defined themselves as black should have felt positive about their racialised identity. The rest could be expected to yearn to be white, or to feel confused about whether they were white or black, and in general to feel unhappy about, and ashamed of, their mixed ancestry. It was in order to see whether or not those beliefs are justified that we addressed the issue of whether or not the young people of mixed parentage in our study had a positive black identity. In fact we found that using fairly stringent criteria, including definite pride in their colour, 60 per cent of the sample had a positive racialised identity, but of this 60 per cent, nearly three-quarters thought of themselves as 'mixed' rather than black. They were proud of their mixed parentage and saw more advantages than disadvantages in it, particularly in their ability to feel comfortable with both black and white people, and to see both their points of view.

Twenty per cent of the sample showed some of the classically 'marginal' characteristics. They wished that they were white, or that they were either black or white, rather than 'mixed'. Some felt that they stood out from both black and white people as different, and some were always uncomfortably aware of their colour. Two felt confused, 'as if I don't have a true identity'. We characterised this 20 per cent of the sample as having a problematic rather than a negative racialised identity, because they all also expressed some positive feelings about their mixed parentage. The remaining 20 per cent we put in an intermediate category. They did not want to be another colour, and were not confused or uncomfortable with their colour, but they were not definitely proud of it. Often they said that colour was not a matter for pride, that they were proud of who they were, rather than of their colour.

Which young people of mixed parentage had a positive racialised identity?

Whilst having a *black* identity was related to holding more politicised views of racism, having a *positive* or *problematic* racialised identity was related to quite different factors. Wanting to be white, our major indicator of a problematic identity, was associated with being strongly affiliated to white people, and, to a lesser extent, having a positive identity was associated with attending a multiracial school. Whether the young people were living with a black parent had no bearing on whether or not they had a positive racialised identity, just as it had no bearing on whether or not they thought of themselves as black. We suspect that a particularly bad or a particularly good relationship with one parent influenced the 'race' which the young person identified with, and we have some evidence that the young person's appearance was another influence on identity, but we do not have systematic evidence on these points.

Whatever happened to the marginal personality?

Only one-fifth of the sample, then, described themselves as experiencing problems with their racialised identity. There are a number of reasons why mixed-parentage people today might view their identity more positively than was probably the case in the past. While racism has by no means disappeared, open manifestations of it are no longer acceptable in many settings. Some areas in London are seen by both black and white youth as free from racialised tension; in these areas multiracial friendships flourish, and references to people's colour are considered 'out of order' (Back, 1991b). Both black and white pupils in a number of multiracial secondary schools (although by no means all) told us that open racism by staff or pupils was not permitted, and did not occur. Some mixed-parentage girls, rather than being stigmatised for their appearance, were admired by both black and white girls for their skin colour and ringlets. These factors, together with the greater liberalisation of white attitudes, the success of the black consciousness movement in the 1960s and 1970s, and the increasing number of black and white unions, make it likely that people of mixed black and white parentage suffer rejection less often now than in the past.

Nonetheless, although only a minority experienced problems with their racialised identity, the proportion who did so was twice as large as was the case of the young people with two black parents. Their problems were those that have always been recognised for people of mixed parentage: a feeling of being 'different', a feeling of being torn between two sets of competing loyalties, and in some cases the experience of hostility from black children as well as white.

Advantages and disadvantages of a black identity

On the basis of the general psychological principle that in order to have self-esteem one must feel comfortable with who one is, we believe it is an advantage for young people to feel positive about their mixed parentage. It is, however, less obvious that it is an advantage for them to have a black identity. The advantage is said to be that a black identity accords with the reality that they are seen as black by white people. This argument, however, confuses two meanings of 'black'. It is true that most, although not all, of the sample would be perceived by white people as black, in the sense of not being white, and as such they did indeed meet with racism, just as did the young people with two black parents. However, because the majority of the mixed-parentage sample *looked* different from the black sample, they would also be seen as distinct from them. In a similar way Asian people may be seen as black (not white), but different from African Caribbeans. While some of the mixed-parentage sample were very dark-skinned, and could have had two black parents, some were identifiably 'mixed', others could have been mistaken for Indians or Pakistanis, and some looked white. Many of the sample were likely to have been seen by white people as 'coloured' or 'half-caste', or in some cases as 'Asian'. An identity as 'brown' or 'mixed' at this level was therefore not at variance with the way they were perceived by others.

A definite advantage to having a black identity is that it provides a large community with which to identify. (This would also be true of identifying with white people, but this option was not open to most of our sample because of their appearance.) A number of the young people in the study, and their parents, mentioned the disadvantage of knowing very few other people of mixed parentage; some tried to convert this into an advantage by seeing themselves as 'very special'. But we found that those mixed-parentage young people in multiracial schools where there were a number of others like themselves tended to say that they felt more comfortable with them than with either black or white students. There are other difficulties in sustaining a mixed identity. Not only are there as yet relatively few mixed-parentage people in Britain, there is also no culture – institutions, history, literature, music, heroes or rituals – that is distinctively their own. Heroes from one's own racialised and/or ethnicised group with whom one can identify play an important role in many people's lives. It was important to Samuel Coleridge-Taylor, the late nineteenth-century mixed-parentage composer, to believe that some of his heroes 'had coloured blood in their veins', and he was convinced that this was the case with Beethoven and Robert Browning (Sayers, 1915: 45, 103). There have, of course, been eminent people of mixed parentage, especially in the USA, but they are not widely known as such, since they are usually simply referred to as 'black'. Official forms do not often invite mixed-parentage people to describe their dual inheritance. Thus, looking into society, they see no reflection or validation of themselves.

However, there are disadvantages to claiming a black identity. Black people do not always accept them as black: a minority of our sample had met hostility, exclusion and verbal abuse from black children. For those who regarded themselves as black this was a disturbing experience, which in some ways parallels the rejection in the last century of mixed-parentage people who tried to 'pass' as white. Further, opting for a black identity entails discounting the white part of one's inheritance. Most (but not all) of the young people's closest attachments were to their mothers, who were generally white. Regarding themselves as black often seemed to them a form of betrayal, or at least rejection, and they preferred to think of themselves as 'half-and-half'. This point is overlooked by those who argue that, since most African Caribbeans are racially mixed, mixed-parentage people differ from them only in the time at which the mix occurred. While this may be true with respect to their genes it is not true psychologically, because of the mixed-parentage child's emotional bond with their white parent. The majority of our sample seemed very confident in their identity as 'both black and white'. Such an identity may be combined with a feeling of solidarity with other black people from a range of groups.

Did the young people bridge black and white cultures?

The young people themselves often claimed as an advantage of their mixed parentage that they could bridge both black and white cultures. However, the reality seemed to be more complex. We did indeed find that two-thirds of the sample said they felt equally comfortable with black and white people, and an even larger proportion said they had no colour preference for a marriage partner. They were certainly more likely than the young white people to have a close friend, and boyfriend or girlfriend, who was black, and much more likely than the young black people to have a close friend, and boyfriend or girlfriend, who was white. In these respects they moved more easily between black and white cultures than did either the black or the white group.

But these overall figures conceal the fact that some of the sample were strongly affiliated to white people and culture, while others were strongly affiliated to black people and culture. Because just over half our sample attended predominantly white schools, and lived in white districts, twice as many young people in the sample had white friends as had black. The girlfriends and boyfriends of those attending predominantly white schools were almost always white, and they usually had no particular liking for the music or clothes of contemporary black youth cultures. They were thus predominantly situated within white cultures. However, the rest of the sample who attended multiracial comprehensive schools lived in a very different racialised and cultural environment. They were much more likely to have close black friends, although all but one had some white friends, not necessarily close friends, as well. They tended to be enthusiastic adherents of some form of contemporary black youth culture, and the public figures they admired were often black.

A minority of the young people had strong affiliations to *both* black *and* white people and cultures – only 30 per cent, for example, had both white and black close friends, and only 30 per cent had had both black and white boyfriends or girlfriends. This was partly because the boundaries between black and white people and their cultures are to some extent also social class boundaries. The black middle class in Britain is still very small, so that the majority of young black people come from working-class families. It is among these young people that black youth culture flourishes. Thus those who had strong ties with both black and white people and their cultures tended to be those who crossed social class as well as racialised boundaries. They might be young people from working-class families attending independent schools, or middle-class young people attending multiracial comprehensive schools, or students at independent schools who lived in a mixed neighbourhood and had a network of black friends. It was not always easy for young people from middle-class families to make these friends because of the tendency of black working-class youth to mistrust them, but those alive to the attraction of black 'style' persevered. As one of them said:

> ''Cos now, you know, fashion sways towards black people. You are better to be black than white, because everyone now respects you even more if you are black. It's funny, really, because it used to be the other way round. It's black people's fashions, the trainers and the jeans, and the people who started it were the black people in New York. They started their own culture, and now it's come over here, but the thing is, white people are doing it as well.'

However, unlike this girl, a substantial proportion of our sample, in both racially mixed and predominantly white schools, had no strong sense of black–white boundaries; that is, of black and white people having distinct characteristics and cultures. Only a quarter, for example, thought that black and white people have different tastes in such matters as music and fashion, the majority arguing that there is a good deal of overlap. Seventy per cent said their colour had never prevented them from doing something they wanted to do. Those who did perceive strong white–black boundaries tended to be those who reported more experience of racism.

Although about half of our mixed-parentage sample had visited the country of origin of their black parent, their ties with these countries were rather weak. Few had black grandparents living in this country who might have helped them to develop such an affiliation. Those who wanted to settle in a country other than Britain had their sights on North America, or sometimes Europe, not Africa or the Caribbean. Very few read magazines or newspapers with Caribbean or African links, although two-thirds liked African or Caribbean food. The great majority thought of themselves as English or British; however, for one-third of the young people this was combined with some feeling of loyalty to their black parent's country of origin. But half said they did not feel loyal to, or patriotic about, any country. These young people felt in some sense excluded by white people from English culture, and from being English. At the same time, they felt no tie with Africa or the Caribbean. The majority of the sample identified most easily with being a 'Londoner'. They saw London as a multiracial city, where they felt at home and relatively secure. But again, there were very divergent attitudes within the sample, with a minority who felt they were loyal, and even patriotic English citizens, and argued that nowadays 'English' had a multiracial meaning.

Racism and family communication

The young people of mixed parentage were slightly more likely to report experiences of racism than those with two black parents. The extent to which they did so varied widely. For a few, racism was a disturbing aspect of daily life. A small number, most of whom looked white, said they had never experienced racism. While the great majority had experienced name-calling in primary school, a quarter of the sample said that had been their only experience of racism. Only one-third said they had been called names in recent years, and this was usually in the street rather than at school. Contrary to what is often believed, racist abuse was reported to be more frequent, and was experienced as much more wounding, in primary than in secondary school.

The extent to which the young people described experiencing racism themselves, and being aware of it within their family and their school (our combined variable of 'experience of racism'), varied widely. Those young people who described a high level of communication about race within the family, and who believed that their parents' views on racism had influenced them, and who held more politicised views on racism, were likely to report more experience of racism, as were those young people for whom race was more central, and who perceived greater boundaries between black and white people and their cultures.

It is not possible to know whether their greater experience of racism led to more family communication about it, or whether their more politicised views and the greater amount of communication about racism sensitised the young people to the presence of racism. It was clear that some were *not* sensitised. Incidents interpreted as racist by some would be ignored or dismissed by others. They might dismiss verbal abuse as joking, attribute being watched in shops or stopped by the police to their youth, and failing to get a job to inexperience rather than to discrimination.

The young people of mixed parentage had the same level of awareness of racism in society (e.g. in employment and housing) as those with two black parents. Those who showed the most awareness of racism in society tended to be more affiliated to black people, and little affiliated to white people.

Racism, gender and class

Racist name-calling, observing racism, and describing racism as present in their school were more often reported by boys and young people from working-class families. Being a mixed-parentage girl in a middle-class girls' school was thus a very different and easier experience from being a mixed-parentage boy in a mainly working-class school. In such schools racialised insults and 'cussing' were often an accepted part of masculine youth culture. This was also the case in some of the boys' independent schools, where the few black or mixed-parentage boys could feel very isolated. While in some contexts mutual racialised insults were seen by the young people as 'joking' or a form of play, they could rapidly escalate into hurtful racist abuse. In contrast, middle-class girls' schools were a relatively safe haven for mixed-parentage girls.

Working-class mixed-parentage boys, like those with two black parents, were liable to suffer not only from racialised abuse but also from the widely held stereotype of the young black male as prone to violence and criminal behaviour. It was not only white people who had absorbed this stereotype; despite having no personal knowledge of them, some of the mixed-parentage middle-class boys and girls were wary, if not fearful, of working-class black male youths.

'Survival skills' and family communication about racism

White parents have been said to be unable to hand on to their children the 'survival skills' needed to cope in a racist society. All the young people in our sample had consciously formulated strategies for dealing with racism, often using a variety of strategies to suit different situations. Ignoring racist incidents, or discounting them as too stupid to bother about, were the most common strategies, and were adopted by all the young people on occasion. A minority chose to tackle racists directly whenever they could, usually by means of counter-insults. Some felt that excelling in any sphere was the best way of minimising the effects of racism. We did not find any differences between the ways in which young people living with a black, or with only white parents, dealt with racism. Nor did the young people's account of the advice given by their parents, which was usually to ignore the incident, or their accounts of the models they provided of dealing with racism, differ according to the colour of the parent.

It is possible that indirect approaches to helping children deal with racism, such as telling them to be proud of their colour (half had been told) and talking to them about famous black people (two-thirds of the parents had done this), are more effective forms of parental support than direct advice. Again, we found no difference in the proportion of young people living with a black parent or with white parents only who said their parents had used these approaches. In only half of the families was there any overt communication about race and racism, whether in the form of advice, discussion of a parent's or child's experience, or general comments. These proportions may seem low, but they are not very different from the proportions reported by the young people with two black parents. One-third of the young people of mixed parentage who had experienced some form of racism had never discussed it with anyone. And half of the parents we interviewed were unaware of, or underestimated, the amount of racism their children said they experienced.

This is not a surprising finding, given that other studies have shown that parents tend to overestimate their children's happiness at school, and underestimate their worries and fears (Lapouse and Monk, 1959; Tizard *et al.*, 1988). In part, the young people, believing that their parents could not help, may have been protecting them from anxiety. But this was not the whole story. We found that the young people's lack of communication tended to be matched by that of their parents. Our interviews with a small sample of parents suggested that in some cases lack of communication was the result of a deliberate policy of 'not making too much' of racism. Another factor was probably involved: the low level of communication in many families on most topics outside the daily round was striking.

Social class, and the racialised composition of school and family

Being of mixed parentage was a different experience for young people from working-class and middle-class families. We have already reported that those from working-class families were more likely to say they experienced racist abuse than those from middle-class families, and more likely to say there was racism in their schools. They were also more likely to be adherents of black youth culture. They were more likely than those from middle-class families to say they felt most comfortable with other people of mixed parentage, perhaps because they knew more of them, or because they were more likely than young middle-class people to have experienced discrimination from both black and white young people. They also tended to refer to themselves as 'half-caste', while young middle-class people more often described themselves as being of 'mixed race'.

It is difficult to separate the influence of social class from that of *the racialised composition of the school*, since young people from working-class families were more likely to attend multiracial schools. Those who attended multiracial schools, like those from working-class families, were more likely than others to be adherents of black youth culture, and to feel most comfortable with others of mixed parentage. They were more often strongly affiliated to black people and culture, and less often strongly affiliated to white. On average, as much racism was reported in multiracial schools as in predominantly white schools. These averages conceal a gender difference. While a lot of racism was reported in most of the predominantly white boys' schools, very little was reported in the predominantly white girls' schools. The averages also conceal the differences between multiracial schools – in some, the young people reported a lot of racism, in others, little or none. There was also a tendency for those young people with a racialised identity which we rated as problematic to attend predominantly white schools.

We have already reported that *the racialised composition of the family* – that is, whether the young people lived with at least one black parent, or with a white single parent, and sometimes a white step-parent – had no relationship to whether they thought of themselves as black, or to how positive they felt about their racialised identity. But the racialised composition of the family was related to other aspects of the young people's behaviour and attitudes in an unexpected way. Those who lived with a black parent were less likely to feel that colour was central in their lives than those who lived with a white parent. They were also more likely to be affiliated to white people and their culture, and less likely to be affiliated to black people and their culture than those living only with a white parent. The explanation for these apparently strange findings seemed to be that the young people in our sample who lived with a black parent were more likely to attend almost entirely white independent schools.

The black parents were particularly, and understandably, concerned for the academic success of their children. For this reason, some had chosen predominantly white schools with a reputation for high academic standards. They may have assumed that they themselves would provide an adequate link with black people and their culture. In some cases, where there was a very strong relationship between the black parent and the child, and when the black parent was determined that the child should feel strong links with African or Caribbean culture, this could occur. But more often the young people became absorbed in the culture of the school, often to the extent of internalising white stereotypes about black male youths, and even white standards of beauty.

For a few, this led to a wish to be white, or to a fear of black working-class youth. Attending predominantly white schools could impose some strain on the young people. Boys in schools where the peer group culture was racist could have a difficult life unless they had both an unusual degree of self-confidence and support from their families. Even in the apparently protected environment of a girls' school, the young people could feel uncomfortably conspicuous.

> 'When I started at school there were just three of us in the school, three black people. And I was very conscious when they gave assemblies on racism, and I would look at X [another black girl] and think, They don't know what they're talking about. And it's like you stick out a mile, everyone knows who you are. You see the teachers on the first day of term, and they eye through the class, and usually, say in the first year, everyone looks the same, small, and baggy school uniform, and the same long hair. And there I was with my hair sticking out everywhere, and their eyes would come back to me, and I would think, Oh, no.'

However, other girls seemed to feel comfortable in similarly predominantly white school environments. Moreover, all the young people, even if they wished that there were more black students, appreciated the education and opportunities they thought these schools provided.

The diversity of experience of mixed-parentage people

It should be clear by now that it is difficult to generalise about the mixed-parentage young people in our study. They had little in common other than having one black and one white parent, and in most cases having experienced some level of racism. Their mixed origins carried a wide range of meanings. Some felt that their mixed parentage made them interestingly unusual, while for others it brought an unpleasant feeling of 'difference'. Some were proud of their mixed parentage, others wished they were either black or white. Some thought of themselves as black, others as 'mixed' or brown. Some reported that they had experienced a great deal of racism, others considered they had met very little. Some had many black friends, and were involved in black youth culture; others lived mainly in white society and culture.

We have shown that the different meanings of their mixed parentage for the young people were related to a wide range of factors. Their gender, social class, the type of school they attended, the extent to which their views on race were politicised, and the amount of family communication about race, were all significantly related to their identities and experiences. But many other factors which we did not assess are probably involved in a complex interaction, including the young people's appearance and the quality of their relationship with each parent, as well as their own and their parents' individual characteristics.

The answers of the mixed-parentage group as a whole to our questions, and the scores we derived from them, were always located between those of the black and the white groups. There was one exception, and that was in their reporting of racism. The mixed-parentage young people reported slightly *more* experience of racism than the young people with two black parents, and had an equal awareness of racism in society – in employment, the police, etc. But their intermediate position on the other scores did not mean that they held intermediate views. It was rather that to each question some young people gave answers similar to those of the black group, and rather more gave answers similar to those of the white group.

Identities are subject to change

In considering the implications of these findings for the young people's future lives, it is important to remember that racialised identities, like other social identities, are not fixed entities. Since identities are formed in social interaction, most psychologists regard them as subject to change throughout the life course. In the case of gender, for example, the girl who is a 'tomboy' as a child may acquire a more traditional 'feminine' identity during adolescence. As mixed-parentage young people encounter new experiences, for example, on leaving school and entering new peer groups, changes in their racialised identities are to be expected. Many of our sample led a protected existence in liberal schools and middle-class areas. Encountering racism as they seek employment is likely to make their racialised identity more salient, and perhaps more problematic. If they move from a white suburb to a multiracial area, those with a 'mixed' identity may choose to think of themselves as black; or, if those who think of themselves as black meet numbers of others of mixed parentage, or learn about the US movement to assert the claims of 'biracial' people, they may shift to a mixed identity.

Such changes can certainly take place in adult life. According to his biographer, (Sayers, 1915: 46), at the age of 21 the composer Samuel Coleridge-Taylor 'had been, and for a few years was still to be, painfully sensitive to the implications of inferiority which his negro derivation implied. But later . . . the timid apologetic attitude was replaced by the

spirit of the apostle and champion, with an infinite faith in the possibilities of the darker sons of the earth.' Brought up by a white parent
and step-parent in an all-white environment, with no positive sense of
his racialised identity, when in his mid-twenties he met black American
musicians, visited the USA, and read Du Bois' *The Souls of Black Folk*.
He regarded this as 'the greatest book I have ever read', and from that
time began a lifelong commitment to furthering the cause of black
people.

In both of these issues – the diversity of the young people's identities
and the fact that they reported change – our findings lend support to
complex theories of identity which view it as plural and dynamic.

Implications for parents

We do not believe that easy recommendations for the parents of mixed-
parentage children emerge from our research, since so much depends on
values and judgements and on what is feasible for particular families,
given their individual characteristics and circumstances. We think it is
important that the young people feel comfortable about their racialised
identity, and that they feel at ease with both black and white people and
cultures. Our research suggests that these aims are more difficult to
attain if the young people attend predominantly white schools, especially if they do not move in a black peer group out of school. On the
other hand, parents may feel that what is most important for their
children is to achieve high educational standards and to enhance their
career prospects.

We believe it is important for young people to feel that they have the
support of their parents in dealing with racism, and to feel reasonably
confident about their own ability to deal with it. In our study those
young people from families where there was more communication
about racism seemed generally to deal with it more confidently than
those where there was little communication. However, parents risk bor-
ing or alienating their children if their concern about racism appears
excessive to their children. Parents who do not hold politicised views
about racism may in any case consider that it is in the child's best
interests not to lay too much emphasis on racism.

We did not find that any particular strategies for dealing with
racism emerged as crucially important, but young people seemed more
confident if they had a range of strategies to call on, including non-
aggressive ways of tackling racism directly. Many of the young people
in our study said they would have been helped by more discussions
about how to deal with racist incidents. Parents themselves may well

be helped by discussion with other parents of mixed-parentage children.

Support for changes in government statistics

A number of young people in our sample told us that they had been upset when filling out official forms at being forced to identify themselves as 'black' or 'white', when they felt themselves to be both or neither. In our study we found no reason for prescribing to an individual that they should identify with a particular group. And since over half our sample opted for a mixed identity, and the size of the mixed population is growing, it seems appropriate that the censuses in both the UK and the USA have now recognised this officially by including 'mixed parentage' in their list of 'ethnic categories'. Clearly the wording used needs to be monitored over time to see if it proves satisfactory, but the initial inclusion would meet with the approval of most of the young people in our study.

Implications for schools

Our study suggested that both individual teachers and school policies could have an important influence on young people's identities. Schools which had a clear and effective antiracist policy seemed to have a positive effect on the day-to-day life and the racialised identities of black and mixed-parentage students. Very real changes had occurred in some secondary schools. Racist remarks by teachers or students which were formerly regular currency would, if they were made now, result in serious disciplinary charges. In schools where racism was not challenged, it seemed more difficult for the young people to sustain a positive identity. Some young people told us that it was a teacher rather than their parents who introduced them to black history, told them about contemporary black leaders, and discussed racism with them. Others we have quoted commented on the important influence that drama and role play at school had on their identity.

Whether teachers should give advice to individual children about how they should define themselves is a different issue. Some young people in our sample who had been advised by teachers to regard themselves as black resented and disregarded this advice. It seems important that schools, like governments, should be aware of the different and legitimate ways in which people of mixed parentage can define themselves, while allowing them to make the decision. There is a case, however, for arguing that schools should help young people to deal with racism, since only half of the young people said they received such help from their parents. But advice is, in any case, difficult to give, and can be taken amiss if the young people do not respect the advisers, or do not believe they are qualified to offer advice. Group discussions, or role play, which involves the group in exchanging their experiences, may be a more effective approach.

The young people in our study described experiencing much more racialised abuse at primary than at secondary school. Schools can act as very effective amplifiers of racialised prejudice. At a young age children are less able to deal with abuse, and find it much more wounding. This suggests that primary schools need to look again at their antiracist policies, which should be at least as thorough, consistent and effective as those in secondary schools. There is now a much greater awareness than in the past of the extent of bullying in primary schools, and the distress this may cause. A number of primary schools have developed effective anti-bullying policies and practices, and similar practices could be used to curb racialised discrimination and taunts, and improve interracial relationships.

Implications for fostering and adoption

A major aim of our study was to examine the assumptions underlying the social work policy that mixed-parentage children in care should be adopted or fostered only by black or racially mixed families. The arguments in favour of this policy are that mixed-parentage children should be regarded as black, since that is how they are seen by society; that if placed in a white family they will not acquire a positive black identity, and will suffer identity confusion; that black people will then reject them for 'not being black enough in culture and attitude'; and that unless very carefully trained, white families will be unable to provide the children with the 'survival techniques' they need to cope in a racist society.

The question of how mixed-parentage people are seen by white society was discussed above. Certainly, those young people in our sample with a 'mixed' identity were under no illusion that this allowed them to escape from racism. They saw themselves rather as another group, who, like Asian people, were subject to racism but who had a different identity from people with two African or African Caribbean parents.

In our study, having a black identity, or a positive identity, was not related to the colour of the parents with whom the young people were growing up. A black identity was related to holding politicised views about racism, while wanting to be white was related to being affiliated in friendships and culture to white people. Affiliation to white people was related to the racialised composition of the school, not the family. A mixed identity was as likely to be positive as a black identity. The young people seemed to have no one set of 'survival skills' for dealing with racism. They used the range of coping mechanisms which all of us use to deal with potentially threatening situations, most frequently ignoring racist abuse or returning it. Some were acquiring the ability to tackle racist situations in direct but non-violent ways, while others would have profited from help in learning these skills. We did not find that the young people growing up with a black parent used different strategies from the others.

We did not find, either, that black parents were transmitting different ways of dealing with racism from those suggested by white parents. According to their children, only half of the parents offered advice about how to deal with racism, or discussed their own experiences of racism, or encouraged the young people to feel proud of their colour, or talked to them about famous black people. Black parents were no more likely to do so than white parents. On the basis of the evidence we have from parents and children it seems likely that those parents, whether black or white, who used these strategies were those with more politicised views of racism.

The question of whether someone is 'black enough in culture and attitude' (Small, 1986: 93) seems to assume that there is a unitary black culture shared by all black people, irrespective of their gender, age, social class or country of origin. In keeping with theories of racialised identities that have been proposed since 1986 when Small published this paper, we do not believe that there is a unitary black culture; what unites black people is rather the experience of racism. In our sample, while all but two of the black parents had grown up in Africa or the Caribbean, most of the young people had been born in England. Only one-third felt any loyalty to their black parent's country of origin, and their ties to it seemed very weak. They saw themselves very much as English, or British, and particularly as Londoners. More than half had some allegiance to one of the contemporary black British youth cultures, which derive from the USA as well as the Caribbean. Allegiance to both Africa or the Caribbean, and to black British youth cultures, was much stronger in young people from working-class families. The young people from middle-class families, whether or not they were living with a black parent, were in the main situated within white English cultures, and tended to have mainly white friends. They spoke in a middle-class English speech style, for preference ate Italian or Chinese food, read the *Independent* or the *Guardian*, and preferred listening to pop or classical music. Nevertheless, they regarded themselves as mixed black or 'half-and-half', not white.

What are the implications of our findings for social work policy? We do not want to suggest that one small-scale research project is an adequate basis in itself for changing policy. We do, however, believe that it raises serious questions about some of the assumptions underlying policy, especially since the findings are consistent with those of most other studies of mixed-parentage children and adolescents who are not 'looked after'. In particular, we believe it is time to reconsider the assumption that mixed-parentage children 'should have' a black identity, and that the colour of the foster or adoptive parents is of paramount importance. It may be objected that because 60 per cent of our sample came from middle-class families, and half attended private schools, the findings are not relevant to the kind of children who enter care. There are two reasons why this objection is mistaken. In the first place the adoption studies, which caused alarm by showing that in most transracial placements the children tend to have white friends, and do not identify strongly with black people and cultures, were mainly concerned with placements in middle-class families. We found similar characteristics in young people in middle-class families who lived with their own parents. They were related, not to the colour of the parents, but to the racialised composition of the schools and neighbourhood. Table 11.1 (see Appendix) shows that young people who attended independent schools were very unlikely to be affiliated to black people and their culture, or to black youth culture, or to have politicised views on racism, but were very likely to be strongly affiliated to white people and their culture.

Second, although we found major social class differences in the experience and attitudes of our sample, there were no social class differences in whether the young people had a black or a 'mixed' or a positive or a problematic identity. The young people from working-class families were more likely to be affiliated to black people and their culture and to have more experience of racism than those from middle-class families, but there were no differences in their racialised identities.

We do not want to suggest that *any* white (or indeed black) person would be an adequate foster or adoptive parent for mixed-parentage young people, or that colour is irrelevant when considering their placement. The 'same-race placement' policy campaign performed an important role in calling attention to the earlier neglect of racialised and ethnicised issues by social work departments. The parents in our study, unlike most adoptive or natural parents, had formed a relationship with a person of another colour and had brought up their child.

Many, although not all, felt positive, even enthusiastic, about their child's mixed inheritance. A larger proportion of them had taught their children to be proud of their colour than has usually been reported in the case of adoptive parents. However, a few children had been upset by racism from white relatives, and two by hostility to white people from black parents.

It would clearly be unacceptable to allow children to be fostered or adopted by people with racist views, or those, whether white or black, who were hostile to, or even unenthusiastic about, one half of the child's inheritance. But our findings suggest that the colour of the parents is likely to have less impact on their child's development than their attitudes towards colour and racism, and their social class.

The ideological standpoint of both parents and young people – that is, whether they hold 'politicised' views of racism – seems of particular significance. Moreover, both our findings and those of McRoy and Zurcher (1983) suggest that the influences on racialised identity are much wider than the family. They include neighbourhood, school, and friendship networks, as well as media and societal attitudes to race and ethnicity. Whatever the colour of their parents, adolescents living in a white suburb, attending a predominantly white school, are likely to have very different identities to those living in a racially mixed area, attending a multiracial school. The social policy context is now one where, unlike when the first edition of this book was published, both British and US governments have legislated for minority ethnic group children to be placed for adoption with white majority parents in preference to spending long periods in care. This makes it even more important that attention is paid to issues of racism and neighbourhood when placement decisions are being made.

Social workers may be surprised at the relative lack of identity problems in the young people in our sample. This is because social workers mainly encounter the small minority of young people whose families experience severe problems, and who may themselves be psychologically disturbed. But the negative attitudes to their colour that may be found in these young people and their white mothers seem to be unusual in studies based on secondary schools and the general community. In these studies, one is more likely to encounter young people and their parents who feel positive about, and even proud of, their mixed parentage. As the number of racially mixed marriages and partnerships grows, these attitudes may increasingly be shared and respected.

Appendix

Statistical tables

Notes

1   KW in the tables stands for Kruskal-Wallis 1-way Anova Chi-Square, corrected for ties, P. for Pearson Chi-Square, Sp.C.C. for Spearman Correlation Coefficient.

2   In some tables one or more variables are composed of the sum of scores to a number of questions. In cases where one or more of these questions were not asked, usually because the interview had to be curtailed, the score could not be given, and the total number (N) is reduced.

Table 5.1 Type of school attended by 58 children (%)

Independent	55	Local authority	45
Predominantly white	59	Multiracial	41
All/mostly single sex	65	Even mix of sexes	36

Note: Boys' schools 27%, girls' schools 38%
Total number of schools: 32

Table 5.2 Social class and origin of parents of 58 children (%)

1 *Social class 1 and 2*	61	*Social class 3, 4 and 5*	39
2 *Mother's origin*		*Mother's origin*	
Britain, Canada, etc.	74	• Caribbean	19
(all but one white)		• African	7
		(all black)	
3 *Father's origin*		*Father's origin*	
Britain, Canada, etc.	31	• Caribbean	43
(all but one white)		• African	26
		(all black)	

Table 5.3 Family structure (58 children) (%)

Mother only	Father only	Parent and step-parent	Both parents	Other relatives
28	2	10	57	3

Table 5.4 Racialised composition of family (58 children) (%)

Two parents, white and black	Single black parent, or black parent and black step-parent	Single white parent, or white parent and white step-parent
60	12	28

Table 6.1 Use of terms (%)

	N = 86 *By black*	N = 58 *By 'mixed'*	N = 98 *By white*
Calls 'mixed' 'black'	30	46	16
Uses 'coloured'	30	43	61
Uses 'half-caste'	67	43	61
Uses 'mixed race'	19	24	3
Uses 'half-caste' and 'mixed race'	5	12	1

Table 6.2 Associations with thinking self 'black'

With more politicised attitudes	K.W. 13.07	p .0003	N = 54

Table 6.3 Associations with holding more politicised attitudes

With more experience of racism	Sp.C.C. .30	p .02	N = 46
With attending a state school	K.W. 5.3	p .02	N = 54

Table 6.4 Wishing to be another colour (%)

	In the past		*At present*	
	At times	*Often*	*At times*	*Often*
Black (N = 87)	16	12	2	0
White (N = 98)	12	2	7	1
Mixed (N = 57)	28	23	12	2

Table 6.5 Associations with wanting to be another colour now

With strength of affiliation to white people:	P. 14.7	p .002	N = 50

Table 6.6 Associations with type of identity

Problematic identity: With parents telling one to be proud	P. 6.9	p .03	N = 56
Positive identity: With attending a multiracial school	P. 5.2	p .07	N = 56

Table 6.7 Associations with centrality of race

With living with white parents	K.W. 7.3	p .007	N = 43
With affiliation to black people	Sp.C.C. .48	p .001	N = 41
With feeling most comfortable with others of mixed parentage	Sp.C.C. .40	p .004	N = 41
With having more experience of racism	Sp.C.C. .39	p .02	N = 37

Table 7.1 Associations with preference for others of mixed parentage

With being working class	K.W. 10.30	p .001	N = 54
With attending multiracial schools	K.W. 8.2	p .004	N = 55
With attending state schools	K.W. 4.4	p .04	N = 55

Table 7.2 Associations with affiliation to black people

With attending multiracial schools	K.W. 14.0	p .000	N = 49
With attending state schools	K.W. 13.2	p .003	N = 49
With living with white parents only	K.W. 4.9	p .03	N = 49
With being influenced by parent	Sp.C.C. .36	p .005	N = 49

Table 7.3 Associations with affiliation to white people

With attending mainly white schools	K.W. 7.4	p .006	N = 51
With attending independent schools	K.W. 5.2	p .02	N = 51
With living with black parent(s)	K.W. 5.5	p .02	N = 51
With not being influenced by parent	Sp.C.C. .43	p .001	N = 51

Table 7.4 Associations with affiliation to black youth cultures

With being working class	K.W. 5.7	p .02	N = 55
With attending multiracial schools	K.W. 8.6	p .003	N = 55
With attending state schools	K.W. 6.7	p .009	N = 55

Table 7.5 Associations with liking African and Caribbean food

With being working class	P. 10.5	p .01	N = 54
With attending multiracial schools	P. 8.5	p .04	N = 54

Table 7.6 Associations with seeing black and white lives and cultures as different

With more experience of racism	Sp.C.C. .58	p .000	N = 43

Table 8.1 Associations with name-calling in the past

With being male	P. 5.0	p .02	N = 58

Table 8.2 Associations with recent name-calling

With being working class	P. 13.2	p .0003	N = 57

Table 8.3 Associations with saying there is racism at school

With being male	P. 6.9	p .009	N = 56
With being working class	P. 3.7	p .05	N = 55

Table 8.4 Association with having observed racism

With being working class	P. 3.8	p .05	N = 54

Table 8.5 Associations with 'more experience of racism' variable

With greater perceived boundaries between black and white	Sp.C.C. .58	p .000	N = 43
With more family communication about race	Sp.C.C. .49	p .001	N = 42
With believing parents have influenced views	Sp.C.C. .35	p .00	N = 49
With feeling colour more central	Sp.C.C. .33	p .02	N = 37
With holding more politicised views on racism	Sp.C.C. .30	p .02	N = 46

Table 8.6 Associations with awareness of societal racism

With affiliation to black people	Sp.C.C. .44	p .001	N = 46
With little affiliation to white people	Sp.C.C. .35	p .007	N = 48

Table 9.1 Associations with extent of family communication about race

With believing parents influence views on race	Sp.C.C. .60	p .000	N = 48
With more experience of racism	Sp.C.C. .49	p .001	N = 42

Table 9.2 Associations with being advised and influenced by parents

With being more affiliated to black people	Sp.C.C. .36	p .005	N = 49
With being less affiliated to white people	Sp.C.C. .43	p .001	N = 51
With more experience of racism	Sp.C.C. .35	p .006	N = 49

Table 11.1 Associations with attending independent schools

With being middle class	P. 16.2	p .000	N = 56
With not being affiliated to black people	KW 13.2	p .000	N = 49
With not being affiliated to black youth cultures	KW 6.7	p .009	N = 55
With not having politicised views on race	KW 5.5	p .02	N = 54
With being more affiliated to white people	KW 5.2	p .02	N = 51
With not being most comfortable with others of mixed parentage	KW 4.4	p .04	N = 55

Bibliography

Ahmad, B. (1990) *Black Perspectives in Social Work.* Birmingham: Venture Press.

Ajayi, J.F. (1965) *Christian Missions in Nigeria 1841–1891.* London: Longmans.

Alexander, R. and Curtis, C. (1996) 'A review of empirical research involving the transracial adoption of African American children'. *Journal of Black Psychology*, 22: 223–235.

Alibhai-Brown, Y. (2001) *Mixed Feelings: The Complex Lives of Mixed-race Britons.* London: The Women's Press

Alibhai-Brown, Y. and Montague, A. (1992) *The Colour of Love.* London: Virago.

Amin, K., Gordon, P. and Richardson, R. (1991) *Race Issues Opinion Survey: Preliminary Findings.* London: Runnymede Trust (11 Princelet Street, London E1 6QH).

Antonovsky, A. (1956) 'Towards a refinement of the "marginal man" concept'. *Social Forces*, 35(1): 57–62.

BAAF (1997) *Focus on Adoption: A Snapshot of Adoption Patterns in England 1995.* London: BAAF.

Babb, L.A. and Laws, R. (2001) Portions excerpted from *Adopting and Advocating for the Special Needs Child: A Guide for Parents and Professionals.* Westport, Conn: Bergin & Garvey [internet site of the Family Tree Inc. accessed 12 May 2001] http://www.homes4kids.org/transrac.htm

Back, L. (1991a) 'Social context and racist name calling: an ethnographic perspective on racist talk within a south London adolescent community'. *European Journal of Intercultural Studies*, 1(3): 19–38.

Back, L. (1991b) 'Youth, racism, and ethnicity in south London', unpublished Ph.D. thesis, University of London.

Back, L. (1996) *New Ethnicities and Urban Culture: Racisms and Multiculture in Young Lives.* London: UCL Press.

Bagley, C. (1990) 'Adoption of native children in Canada', in R. Simon and H. Alstein (eds), *Transracial Adoption in Different Societies.* New York: Praeger.

Bagley, C. (1993) 'Transracial adoption in Britain: a follow-up study, with policy considerations'. *Child Welfare*, 72(3): 285–299.

Bagley, C. and Young, L. (1979) 'The identity, adjustment, and achievement of transracially adopted children: a review and empirical report', in G.K. Verma and C. Bagley (eds) *Race, Education, and Identity*. London: Macmillan, pp. 192–219.

Banks, N. (1992) 'Mixed-up kid'. *Social Work Today*, 24(3): 12–13.

Banks, N. (1995) 'Children of black mixed parentage and their placement needs'. *Adoption and Fostering*, 19(2): 19–24.

Banks, N. (1996) 'Young single white mothers with black children'. *Clinical Child Psychology and Psychiatry*, 1(1): 19–28.

Banks, N. (1999a) 'Transracial placement outcomes and assessment of racial sensitivity in white carers'. *Educational and Child Psychology*, 16(3): 55–67.

Banton, M. (1977) *The Idea of Race*. London: Tavistock.

Barker, A.J. (1978) *The African Link*, London: Frank Cass.

Barn, R. (1993) *Black Children in the Public Care System*. London: Batsford/ BAAF.

Barn, R. (1999) 'White mothers, mixed-parentage children and child welfare'. *British Journal of Social Work*, 29(2): 269–284.

Barn, R., Sinclair, R. and Ferdinand, D. (1997) *Acting on Principle: An Examination of Race and Ethnicity in Social Services Provision for Children and Families*. London: BAAF.

Bartholet, E. (1994) 'Race matching in adoption: An American perspective', in I. Gaber and J. Aldridge (eds), *In the Best Interests of the Child: Culture, Identity and Transracial Adoption*. London: Free Association Books, pp. 151–187.

Bath, L. and Farrell, P. (1996) 'The attitudes of white secondary school students towards ethnic minorities'. *Educational and Child Psychology*, 13(3): 5–13.

Bebbington, A. and Miles, J. (1989) 'The background of children who enter local authority care'. *British Journal of Social Work*, 19: 349–368.

Beishon, S., Modood, T. and Virdee, S. (1998), *Ethnic Minority Families*. London: Policy Studies Institute.

Benson, S. (1981) *Ambiguous Ethnicity*. Cambridge: Cambridge University Press.

Berrington, A. (1994) 'Marriage and family formation among the white and ethnic minority populations in Britain'. *Ethnic and Racial Studies*, 17(3): 517–546.

Berrington, A. (1996) 'Marriage patterns and inter-ethnic unions', in D. Coleman and J. Salt (eds), *Ethnicity in the 1991 Census. Volume 1: Demographic Characteristics of the Ethnic Minority Populations*. London: HMSO.

Berthoud, R. (1999) *Young Caribbean Men and the Labour Market: A Comparison with Other Ethnic Groups*. York: Joseph Rowntree Foundation.

Berthoud, R. (2001) *Family Formation in Multi-cultural Britain: Three Patterns of Diversity*. University of Essex: Institute for Social and Economic Research.

Berzon, J.R. (1978) *Neither White Nor Black, The Mulatto Character in American Fiction.* New York: New York University Press.

Boulton, M.J. and Smith, P. (1992) 'Ethnic preferences and perceptions among Asian and white British middle school children'. *Social Development,* 1(1): 55–66.

Bowles, D. (1993) 'Bi-racial identity: children born to African-American and white couples'. *Clinical Social Work Journal,* 21(4): 417–428.

Brah, A. (1996) *Cartographies of Diaspora: Contesting Identities.* London: Routledge.

Butt, J. and Mirza, K. (1997) *Social Care and Black Communities.* London: HMSO.

Chambers, H. (1989) 'Cutting through the dogma'. *Social Work Today,* 21(6): 115.

Clark, K.B. (1963) *Prejudice and Your Child.* Boston, MA: Beacon Press.

Clark, K.B. and Clark, M.K. (1939) 'The development of consciousness of self and the emergence of racial identity in Negro preschool children. *Journal of Social Psychology,* 10: 591–599.

Clark, K.B. and Clark, M.K. (1947) 'Racial identification and preference in Negro children', in T. Newcomb and E. Hartley (eds), *Readings in Social Psychology.* New York: Holt, Rinehart and Winston, pp. 169–178.

Cohen, P. (1988) 'Perversions of inheritance: studies in the making of multi-racist Britain', in P. Cohen and H. Bains (eds), *Multi-Racist Britain.* London: Macmillan.

Cohen, P. (1994) 'Yesterday's words, tomorrow's world: from the racialisation of adoption to the politics of difference', in I. Gaber and J. Aldridge (eds), *In the Best Interests of the Child: Culture, Identity and Transracial Adoption.* London: Free Association Books.

Coleman, D. (1985) 'Ethnic intermarriage in Great Britain'. *Population Trends,* 40: 4–10.

Collins, P.H. (1990) *Black Feminist Thought.* Cambridge, MA: Unwin Hyman.

Collins, S. (1957) *Coloured Minorities in Britain.* Guildford: Lutterworth Press.

Commission for Racial Equality (1985) *Birmingham Local Education Authority and Schools: Referral and Suspension of Pupils.* London: CRE.

Commission for Racial Equality (1988) *Medical School Admissions: Report of a Formal Investigation.* London: CRE.

Cunningham, J. (1997) 'Colored existence: racial identity formation in light-skin blacks'. *Smith College Studies in Social Work,* 67(3): 375–400.

Davey, A.G. and Norburn, M.V. (1980) 'Ethnic awareness and ethnic differentiations amongst primary school children'. *New Community,* 8(112): 51–60.

Department of Education and Science (1991) 'Independent schools in England'. *Statistical Bulletin,* January 1990.

Department of Health (1999) *Adoption Now: Messages from Research.* London: Department of Health.

Department of Health (2000) *Adopting Changes Survey and Inspection of Local Councils' Adoption Services*. London: Department of Health.

Dover, C. (1937) *Half Caste*. London: Secker & Warburg.

Durojaiye, M.O.A. (1970) 'Patterns of friendship choice in an ethnically mixed junior school'. *Race*, 13(2): 189–200.

Early Years Trainers Anti-Racist Network (EYTARN) (1995) *The Best of Both Worlds: Celebrating Mixed Parentage*. London: EYTARN.

Economist, The (2001) 'Primary Colours'. 17 March.

Erikson, E.H. (1968) *Identity, Youth and Crisis*. New York: Norton.

Essed, P. (1996) '"As long as they don't call me a racist": Ethnization in the social services', in P. Essed, *Diversity: Gender, Color and Culture*. Amherst: University of Amherst Press.

Fanon, F. (1967) *The Wretched of the Earth*. Harmondsworth: Penguin.

Fatimilehin, I. (1999) 'Of jewel heritage: racial socialization and racial identity attitudes amongst adolescents of mixed African-Caribbean/White parentage'. *Journal of Adolescence*, 22: 303–318.

Feigelman, W. (2000) 'Adjustments of transracially and inracially adopted young adults'. *Child and Adolescent Social Work Journal*, 17(3): 165–183.

Feigelman, W. and Silverman, A. (1983) *Chosen Children: New Patterns of Adoptive Relationships*. New York: Praeger.

Field, L. (1996) 'Piecing together the puzzle: self-concept and the group identity in biracial black/white youth,' in M. Root (ed.), *The Multiracial Experience: Racial Borders as the New Frontier*. Thousand Oaks, CA: Sage.

Fine, M., Powell, L., Weis L. and. Mun Wong , L. (eds) (1997) *Off White*. New York: Routledge.

Foucault, M. (1980) *Power/Knowledge*. Brighton: Harvester Press.

Frankenberg, R. (1993a) *White Women, Race Matters*. London: Routledge.

Frankenberg, R. (1993b) 'Growing up white: feminism, racism and the social geography of childhood'. *Feminist Review*, 45: 51–84.

Frosh, S., Phoenix, A. and Pattman, R. (2001) *Young Masculinities: Understanding Boys in Contemporary Society*. London: Palgrave Press.

Fryer, P. (1984) *Staying Power, The History of Black People in Britain*. London: Pluto Press.

Gaber, I. and Aldridge, J. (eds) (1994) *In the Best Interests of the Child: Culture, Identity and Transracial Adoption*. London: Free Association Books.

Gallup Polls Ltd (1958) No. 2577, September.

Gaskins, P.F. (1999) *What Are You? Voices of Mixed-Race Young People*. New York: Henry Holt.

Gates, H.L. (1994) *Colored People*. Harmondsworth: Penguin.

Gibbs, J. and Hines, A. (1992) 'Negotiating ethnic identity', in M. Root (ed.), *Racially Mixed People in America*. London: Sage, pp. 223–238.

Gill, O. and Jackson, B. (1983) *Adoption and Race*. London: Batsford.

Gilroy, P. (1987) *There Ain't no Black in the Union Jack*. London: Hutchinson.

Gilroy, P. (1994) 'Roots and routes: black identity as an outernational project', in H. Harris, H. Blue and E. Griffith (eds), *Racial **and** Ethnic*

Identity: Psychological development **and** *creative expression*. New York: Routledge.

Gilroy, P. (1996) 'Revolutionary conservatism and the tyrannies of unanimism'. *New Formations*, 28: 65–84.

Gist, N.P. and Dworkin, A.G. (1972) *The Blending of Races: Marginality and Identity in World Perspective*. New York: John Wiley & Sons.

Goldstein, B.P. (1999) 'Black, with a white parent, a positive and achievable identity'. *British Journal of Social Work*, 29(2): 285–301.

Grove, K.J. (1991) 'Identity development in interracial, Asian white late adolescents – must it be so problematic'. *Journal of Youth and Adolescence*, 20(6): 617–628.

Grow, L. and Shapiro, D. (1974) *Black Children – White Parents: A Study of Transracial Adoption*. Washington, DC: Child Welfare League of America.

Hall, A. (1996) *Mixed Race Relationships in the UK*. Warwick: Centre for Research in Ethnic Relations.

Hall, S. (1992) 'Questions of cultural identity', in S. Hall, D. Held and T. McGrew (eds), *Modernity and its Futures*. Cambridge: Polity Press.

Hall, S. (1996) 'Introduction: who needs "identity"?', in S. Hall and P. du Gay (eds), *Questions of Cultural Identity*. London: Sage, pp. 1–17.

Haskey, J. (1991) 'The ethnic minority populations resident in private households – estimates by county and metropolitan districts of England and Wales'. *Population Trends*, 63 (spring): 22–35.

Haugaard, J. (2000) 'Research and policy on transracial adoption: comments on Park and Green'. *Adoption Quarterly*, 3(4): 35–41.

Hayes, P. (1993) 'Transracial adoption: politics and ideology'. *Child Welfare*, 72: 301–310.

Heaton, T.B. and Albrecht, S.L. (1996) 'The changing patterns of international marriage'. *Social Biology*, 43(3–4): 203–217.

Henwood, K. and Phoenix, A. (1996) '"Race" in psychology: teaching the subject'. *Ethnic and Racial Studies*, 19(4): 841–863.

Heron, L. (ed.) (1985) *Truth, Dare or Promise, Girls Growing Up in the Fifties*. London: Virago.

Herring, R. (1995) 'Developing biracial ethnic identity: a review of the increasing dilemma'. *Journal of Multicultural Counseling and Development*, 23: 29–38.

Hewitt, R. (1986) *White Talk Black Talk: Inter-racial Friendship and Communication Amongst Adolescents*. Cambridge: Cambridge University Press.

Hollingsworth, L. (1997) 'Effect of transracial/transethnic adoption on children's racial and ethnic identity and self-esteem: a meta-analytic review'. *Marriage and Family Review*, 25(1/2): 99–130.

Hollingsworth, L. (1998) 'Adoptee dissimilarity from the adoptive family: clinical practice and research implications'. *Child and Adolescent Social Work Journal*, 15(4): 303–319.

Holmes, R. (1995) *How Young Children Perceive Race*. Thousand Oaks, CA: Sage.

Hoyles, A. and Hoyles, M. (1999) *Remember Me*. London: Hansib Publications.

Hutnik, N. (1991) *Ethnic Minority Identity: A Social Psychological Perspective*. Oxford: Oxford Science.

Huxley, J.S. (1936) 'Eugenics and society'. *Eugenics Review*, 38: 11–31.

Ifekwunigwe, J. (1997) 'Diaspora's daughters, Africa's orphans? On lineage, authenticity and "mixed race" identity', in H.S. Mirza (ed.), *Black British Feminism: A Reader*. London: Routledge.

Ifekwunigwe, J. (1999) *Scattered Belongings: Cultural Paradoxes of 'Race', Nation and Culture*. London: Routledge.

ILEA (1983) *Race, Sex and Class, 2: Multiethnic Education in Schools*. Appendix B.

Ivaldi, G. (2000) *Surveying Adoption: A Comprehensive Analysis of Local Authority Adoptions 1998/1999 – England*. London: BAAF.

Jackson, J., McCullough, W. and Gurin, G. (1986) 'Family, socialization environment, and identity development in Black Americans', in H.P. McAdoo (ed.), *Black Families: Second Edition*. Newbury Park, CA: Sage.

James, J. (1997) 'The views and perceptions of environmental and public health issues for children from different ethnic communities living in Stepney and Wapping'. Paper presented to a Department of Health Conference *The Health and Health Care of Children and Young People from Minority Ethnic Groups in Britain*. London: National Children's Bureau, 23–24 January.

Jones, A. and Butt, J. (1995) *Taking the Initiative*. London: NSPCC

Jones, R.S. (1994) 'The end of Africanity: The bi-racial assault on blackness'. *The Western Journal of Black Studies*, 18(4): 201–210.

Jones, S. (1988) *White Youth, Black Culture: The Reggae Tradition from JA to UK*. Basingstoke: Macmillan.

Jones, S. (1991) The Reith Lecture. *Independent*, 12 December.

Kahn, J. and Denmon, J. (1997) 'An examination of social science literature pertaining to multiracial identity; a historical perspective'. *Journal of Multicultural Social Work*, 6(1/2): 117–138.

Katz, I. (1995) 'Anti-racism and modernism', in M. Yelloly and M. Henkel (eds), *Learning and Teaching in Social Work: Towards Reflective Practice*. London: Jessica Kingsley.

Katz, I. (1996) *The Construction of Racial Identity in Children of Mixed Parentage: Mixed Metaphors*. London: Jessica Kingsley.

Kelly, C. and Breinlinger, S. (1996) *The Social Psychology of Collective Action*. London: Falmer Press.

Kerwin, C., Ponterotto, J., Jackson, B. and Harris, A. (1993) 'Racial identity in biracial children: a qualitative investigation'. *Journal of Counseling Psychology*, 40(2): 221–231.

Khan, Y. (in prep.) *Beyond Black or White: Mixed Race Britons*. London: Routledge.

Kim, S.P., Hong, S. and Kim, B.S. (1979) 'Adoption of Korean children by New York couples'. *Child Welfare*, 58: 419–427.

Kirton, D. (1995) *'Race', Identity and the Politics of Adoption*. University of East London Centre for Adoption and Identity Studies, Working Paper no. 2.

Kirton, D. (1996) 'Review Article: Race and adoption'. *Critical Social Policy*, 16(1): 123–136.

Kirton, D. (1999) 'Perspectives on "race" and adoption: The views of student social workers'. *British Journal of Social Work*, 29(5): 779–796.

Korgen, K. (1998) *From Black to Biracial: Transforming Racial Identity Among Americans*. Westport, CT: Praeger.

Lampe, P.E. (1978) 'Ethnic self-referent and the assimilation of Mexican Americans'. *International Journal of Comparative Sociology*, 19: 259–270.

Lapouse, R. and Monk, M.A. (1959) 'Fears and worries in a representative sample of children'. *American Journal of Orthopsychiatry*, 29: 803–818.

Lewis, G. (1996) 'Black women's experience and social work'. *Feminist Review*, 53: 24–56.

Lewis, G. (2000) *'Race', Gender, Social Welfare: Encounters in a Postcolonial Society*. Cambridge: Polity Press.

Little, K. (1948) *Negroes in Britain*. London: Routledge & Kegan Paul.

Luke, C. and Luke, A. (1998) 'Interracial families: difference within difference'. *Ethnic and Racial Studies*, 21(4): 728–755.

Luke, C. and Luke, A. (1999) 'Theorizing interracial families and hybrid identity: an Australian perspective'. *Educational Theory*, 49(2): 223–249.

McBride, J. (1998) *The Color of Water: A Black Man's Tribute to His White Mother*. London: Bloomsbury.

Macdonald, I., Bhavnani, R., Khan, L. and John, G. (1989) *Murder in the Playground*. London: Longsight Press.

Mackey, H. (1972) 'The complexion of the accused: William Davidson, the black revolutionary'. *Negro Educational Review*, 23: 132–147.

McRoy, R. (1994) 'Attachment and racial identity issues: implications for child placement decision making'. *Journal of Multicultural Social Work*, 3(3): 59–74.

McRoy, R. and Grape, H. (1999) 'Skin color in transracial and inracial adoptive placements: implications for special needs adoptions'. *Child Welfare*, 78(5): 673–692.

McRoy, R.G. and Zurcher, L.A. (1983) *Transracial and Inracial Adoptees*. Springfield, IL: Charles C. Thomas.

Majors, R. and Billson, J (1992) *Cool Pose: The Dilemmas of Black Manhood in America*. New York: Simon & Schustar.

Mama, A. (1995) *Beyond the Masks: Race, Gender and Subjectivity*. London: Routledge.

Maxime, I.E. (1986) 'Some psychological models of black self-concept', in S. Ahmed, J. Cheetham and I. Small (eds), *Social Work with Black Children and their Families*. London: Batsford, pp. 100–116.

Miles, R. (1989) *Racism*. London: Routledge.

Milner, D. (1983) *Children and Race Ten Years On*. London: Ward Lock Educational.

Modood, T. (1988) ' "Black", racial equality and Asian identity'. *New Community*, 14(3): 397–404.

Modood, T. (1997) 'Culture and identity', in T. Modood, R. Berthoud, J. Lakey, J. Nazroo, P. Smith, S. Virdee and S. Beishon, *Ethnic Minorities in Britain: Diversity and Disadvantage*. London: Policy Studies Institute.

Modood, T., Beishon, S. and Virdee, S. (1994) *Changing Ethnic Identities*. Policy Studies Institute.

Modood, T., Berthoud, R., Lakey, J., Nazroo, J., Smith, P., Virdee, S. and Beishon, S. (1997) *Ethnic Minorities in Britain: Diversity and Disadvantage*. Policy Studies Institute.

Montemayor, R. and Eisen, M. (1977) 'The development of self conceptions from childhood to adolescence'. *Developmental Psychology*, 13(4): 314–319.

Morrison, J.W. (1995) 'Developing identity formation and self-concept in preschool-aged biracial children'. *Early Child Development and Care*, 111: 141–152.

Murphy, J., John, M. and Brown, H. (1983) *Dialogues and Debates in Social Psychology*. London: Lawrence Erlbaum.

National Adoption Information Clearinghouse (2001) Adoption statistics – a brief overview [internet accessed 11 May] http://calib.com/naic/pubs/s_over.htm

Norment, L. (1995) 'Am I black, white or in between? Is there a plot to create a "colored" buffer race in America?' *Ebony*, August, pp. 108–112.

Oden, C. and MacDonald, W.S. (1983) 'Comment: the RIP [reasonable inferential process] in social scientific reporting', in S. Scarr, *Race, Social Class, and Individual Differences in IQ*. London: Lawrence Erlbaum, pp. 149–155.

Ogilvy, C., Boath, E., Cheyne, W., Jahoda, G. and Schaffer, H.R. (1990) 'Staff attitudes and perceptions in multi-cultural nursery schools'. *Early Child Development and Care*, 64: 1–13.

Ogilvy, C., Boath, E., Cheyne, W., Jahoda, G. and Schaffer, H.R. (1992) 'Staff–child interaction styles in multi-ethnic nursery schools'. *British Journal of Developmental Psychology*, 10: 85–97.

Omi, M. and Winant, H. (1986) *Racial Formation in the United States: From the 1960s to the 1980s*. New York: Routledge & Kegan Paul.

OPCS (1992) *General Household Survey – 1991*. London: HMSO.

Owen, C. (1993) 'Using the Labour Force Survey to estimate Britain's ethnic minority populations'. *Population Trends*, 72: 18–23.

Owen, C. (2001) ' "Mixed race" in official statistics', in D. Parker and M. Song (eds) *Rethinking 'Mixed Race'*. London: Pluto Press.

Owen, D. (1994) *Ethnic Minority Women and the Labour Market: Analysis of the 1991 Census*. Manchester: Equal Opportunities Commission.

Park, R. (1928) 'Human migration and the marginal man'. *American Journal of Sociology*, 33: 881–893.

Park, R. (1931) 'The mentality of racial hybrids'. *American Journal of Sociology*, 36: 534–551.

Park, S. and Green, C.E. (2000) 'Is transracial adoption in the best interests of ethnic minority children?: Questions concerning legal and scientific interpretations of a child's best interests'. *Adoption Quarterly*, 3(4): 5–34.

Patterson, S. (1963) *Dark Strangers*. London: Tavistock.

Phinney, J. and Rosenthal, D. (1992) 'Ethnic identity in adolescence: process, context, and outcome', in G. Adams, T. Gullotta and R. Montemayor (eds), *Adolescent Identity Formation*. London: Sage, pp. 145–172.

Phinney, J., Lochner, B. and Murphy, R. (1990) 'Ethnic identity development and psychological adjustment in adolescence', in A. Stiffman and L. Davis (eds), *Ethnic Issues in Adolescent Mental Health*. Newbury Park, CA: Sage.

Phoenix, A. (1987) 'Theories of gender and black families', in G. Weiner and M. Arnot (eds), *Gender Under Scrutiny*. London: Hutchinson.

Phoenix, A. (1997) ' "I'm white so what?" The construction of whiteness for young Londoners', in M. Fine, L. Powell, L. Weis and L. Mun Wong (eds), *Off White*. New York: Routledge, pp. 187–197.

Phoenix, A. (1998) ' "Multicultures", "multiracisms" and young people: contradictory legacies of "Windrush" '. *Soundings*, 10: 86–96.

Phoenix, A. and Owen, C. (1996/2000) 'From miscegenation to hybridity: mixed parentage and mixed relationships in context', in J. Brannen and B. Bernstein (eds), *Children, Research and Policy*. London: Taylor & Francis. Reprinted in A. Brah and A. Coombes (2000) *From Miscegenation to Hybridity*. London: Routledge, pp. 111–135/72–95.

Provine, W.B. (1973) 'Geneticists and the biology of race crossing'. *Science*, 182: 790–796.

Qian, Z.C. (1997) 'Breaking the racial barriers: variations in interracial marriage between 1980 and 1990'. *Demography*, 34(2): 263–276.

Quinton, D., Rushton, A., Dance, C. and Mayes, D. (1998) *Joining New Families: A Study of Adoption and Fostering in Middle Childhood*. Chichester: John Wiley.

Ramdin, R. (1987) *The Making of the Black Working Class in Britain*. Aldershot: Wildwood House.

Rattansi, A. and Phoenix, A. (1998) 'Rethinking youth identities: modernist and postmodernist frameworks', in J. Bynner, L. Chisholm and A. Furlong (eds), *Youth, Citizenship and Social Change in a European Context*. Aldershot: Ashgate, pp. 121–150.

Rhodes, P.J. (1992) 'The emergence of a new policy: racial matching in fostering and adoption'. *New Community*, 18(2): 191–208.

Richards, W. (1995) 'Working with "mixed race" young people'. *Youth and Policy*: 62–72.

Richmond, A. (1961) *The Colour Problem*. Harmondsworth: Penguin.

Root, M. (1992) 'Back to the drawing board: methodological issues in research on multiracial people', in M. Root (ed.), *Racially Mixed People in America*. London: Sage, pp. 181–189.

Root, M. (1996) 'The multiracial experience: racial borders as a significant frontier in race relations,' in M. Root (ed.), *The Multiracial Experience: Racial Borders as the New Frontier*. Thousand Oaks, CA: Sage.

Root, M. (1998) 'Experiences and processes affecting racial identity development: preliminary results from the biracial sibling project'. *Cultural Diversity and Mental Health*, 4(3): 237–247.

Root, M. (2001) *Love's Revolution: Interracial Marriage*. Philadelphia, PA: Temple University Press.

Rose, E.J.B. and associates (1969) *Colour and Citizenship: A Report on British Race Relations*. London: Oxford University Press.

Rosenblatt, P. (1999) 'Multiracial families', in M. Lamb (ed.), *Parenting and Development in 'Nontraditional' Families*. Princeton, NJ: Lawrence Erlbaum.

Rowe, J., Hundleby, M. and Garnett, L. (1989) *Child Care Now*. London: British Agencies for Adoption and Fostering.

Rushton, A. and Minnis, H. (1997) 'Annotation: transracial family placements'. *Journal of Child Psychology and Psychiatry*, 38(2): 147–159.

Saenz, R., Hwang, S.S., Aguirre, B.E. and Anderson, R.N. (1995) 'Persistence and change in Asian identity among children of intermarried couples'. *Sociological Perspectives*, 38(2): 175–194

Sayers, W.C.B. (1915) *Samuel Coleridge-Taylor, Musician: His Life and Times*. London: Cassell and Company.

Scarr, S. and Weinberg, R. (1976) 'IQ test performance of black children adopted by white families', in S. Scarr (ed.) (1983), *Race, Social Class and Individual Differences in IQ*. London: Lawrence Erlbaum Associates.

Schaeffer, N.C. (1980) 'Evaluating race of interviewers effects in a national survey'. *Sociological Methods and Research*, 8: 400–419.

Seacole, M. (1984) *The Wonderful Adventures of Mrs Seacole in Many Lands, 1857* (2nd edition, edited by Ziggi Alexander and Audrey Dewjee). Bristol: Falling Wall Press.

Secretary of State for Health (2000) *Adoption: A New Approach*. A White Paper presented to Parliament by the Secretary of State for Health by Command of Her Majesty Cm 5017, December.

Shyllon, F. (1977) *Black People in Britain, 1555–1833*. Oxford: Oxford University Press.

Silverman, A. (1993) 'Outcomes of transracial adoption'. *Adoption*, 3(1): 104–118.

Simon, R. (1994) 'Transracial adoption: the American experience', in I. Gaber and J. Aldridge (eds), *In the Best Interests of the Child: Culture, Identity and Transracial Adoption*. London: Free Association Books.

Simon, R. and Alstein, H. (1977) *Transracial Adoption*. New York: Wiley-Interscience.

Simon, R. and Alstein, H. (1981) *Transracial Adoption: A Follow-Up*. Lexington, MA: Lexington Books.

Simon, R. and Alstein, H. (1987) *Transracial Adoptees and Their Families: A Study of Identity and Commitment*. New York: Prager.

Simon, R. and Alstein, H. (1996) 'The case for transracial adoption'. *Children and Youth Services Review*, 18(1/2): 5–22.

Simon, R. and Alstein, H. (2000) *Adoption Across Borders: Serving the Children in Transracial and Intercountry Adoptions*. Lanham, MD: Rowan & Littlefield.

Simon, R., Alstein, H. and Melli, M. (1994) *The Case for Transracial Adoption*. Washington, DC: American University Press.

Small, J.W. (1984) 'The crisis in adoption'. *International Journal of Social Psychiatry*, 30(1/2): 129–42.

Small, J.W. (1986) 'Transracial placements: conflicts and contradictions', in S. Ahmed, J. Cheetham and J. Small (eds), *Social Work with Black Children and their Families*. London: Batsford, pp. 81–99.

Spencer, M.B. (1990) 'Development of minority children: an introduction'. *Child Development*, 61(2): 267–269.

Spickard, P. (1989) *Mixed Blood*. Madison: University of Wisconsin Press.

Spickard, P. (1992) 'The illogic of American racial categories', in M. Root (ed.), *Racially Mixed People in America*. Thousand Oaks, CA: Sage.

Stanhope, J. (1962) *The Cato Street Conspiracy*. London: Jonathan Cape.

Stonequist, E.V. (1937) *The Marginal Man: A Study of Personality and Culture Conflict*. New York: Russell and Russell.

Thoburn, J. and Moffatt, P. (2001) 'Outcomes of permanent family placement for children of minority ethnic origin'. *Child and Family Social Work*, 6(1): 13–22.

Thoburn, J., Norford, L. and Rashid, S.P. (2000) *Permanent Family Placement for Children of Minority Ethnic Origin*. London: Jessica Kingsley.

Tizard, B. (1991) 'Intercountry adoption, a review of the evidence'. *Journal of Child Psychology and Psychiatry*, 32: 743–756.

Tizard, B., Blatchford, P., Burke, J., Farquhar, C. and Plewis, I. (1988) *Young Children at School in the Inner City*. Hove and London: Lawrence Erlbaum.

Troyna, B. and Hatcher, R. (1992) *Racism in Children's Lives: A Study of Mainly-White Primary Schools*. London: Routledge.

Twine, F.W. (1996) 'Brown skinned white girls: class, culture and the construction of white identity in suburban communities'. *Gender, Place and Culture*, 3(2): 205–224.

Twine, F.W. (1999a) 'Bearing blackness in Britain: the meaning of racial difference for white birth mothers of African-descent children'. *Social Identities*, 5(2): 185–210.

Twine, F.W. (1999b) 'Transracial mothering and antiracism: the case of white birth mothers of "Black" children in Britain'. *Feminist Studies*, 25(3): 729–746

Twine, F.W. (2001) 'Transgressive women and transracial mothers: white women and critical race theory'. *Meridians*, 1(2): 130–153.

Ullah, P. (1985) 'Second generation Irish youth: identity and ethnicity'. *New Community*, 12: 310–320.

UNESCO (1951) *The Race Concept*. Paris: UNESCO.

Utting, W.B. (1990) *Issues of Race and Culture in the Family: Placement of Children*. Circular CI [90] 2, London: Social Services Inspectorate, Department of Health.

Walker, F.D. (1929) *Thomas Birch Freeman, Son of an African*. London: Student Christian Movement.

Walvin, J. (1973) *Black and White: The Negro and English Society, 1555–1945*. London: Allen Lane.

Webb, J. (1998) 'Racial incidents and mixed race families: a police perspective'. Families' summary of a paper presented to the Institute for Public Policy Research Seminar, 20 March. London: IPPR.

Weekes, D. (1997) *Understanding Young Black Female Subjectivity*. Unpublished Ph.D. thesis, Nottingham Trent University.

Williams, P. (1997) *Seeing a Color-Blind Future: The 1997 Reith Lectures*. London: Noonday.

Williams, T. (1996) 'Race as process: reassessing the "What are You?" encounters of biracial individuals', in M. Root (ed.), *The Multiracial Experience: Racial Borders as the New Frontier*. Thousand Oaks, CA: Sage.

Wilson, A. (1987) *Mixed Race Children: A Study of Identity*. London: Allen and Unwin.

Wright, C. (1992) *Race Relations in the Primary School*. London: David Fulton.

Young, R. (1995) *Colonial Desire: Hybridity in Theory, Culture and Race*. London: Routledge.

Zack, N. (1993) *Race and Mixed Race*. Philadelphia, PA: Temple University Press.

Index

260   *Index*

state schools: survey sample 91;
  working class families 120, 129,
  138
stereotypes: racism 29, 32, 35–6, 148–9
stigma: adoption 56; illegitimacy 27;
  mixed marriages 3; racial mixing 3,
  13, 35
Stonequist, Everett 44, 48

teachers: black teachers 112–13;
  dealing with racism 183–5, 235;
  whether racist 147, 148; white
  teachers 112
terminology: African Americans 7,
  10; Afro-American 10; Asian
  people 12; biracial 9, 10; black 7,
  10, 11, 12, 73, 94, 95, 99, 100, 221;
  black mixed parentage 11; black
  people 12; black with one white
  parent 11; brown 95, 96, 100;
  coloured 7, 8, 10, 94, 95, 96, 100;
  disputes 7–10, 12; dual heritage
  10, 11; ethnic group 5, 13;
  ethnicity 7; half-and-half 95, 238;
  half-breed 3, 11; half-castes 3, 9, 10,
  11, 12, 44, 98–101, 221; insulting
  see insults; intermarriage 9;
  LatiNegra 11; maroon 9;
  mestiza(o) 11; *métis(se)* 3, 9, 11,
  12;miscegenation 9, 10, 12; mixed
  95; mixed breed 3; mixed heritage
  10; mixed marriages 9; mixed
  parentage 10, 11, 12, 98, 219; mixed
  race 9, 12, 57, 98, 99, 100, 221;
  mongrel 11; mulattos 3, 9, 10; negro
  7, 99, 221; nigger 11; race 7, 12, 13;
  racialisation 6, 8, 10, 13; racism 7;
  shift over time 7, 12
Thackeray, William Makepeace 19,
  26, 27, 31
Thatcher, Margaret 125
Thomas, Clarence 74–5
transracial adoption *see* adoption
Tree, Ellen 31

UNESCO 34–5
United States: adoption 57, 58, 60, 80;
  African Americans 7, 10, 23, 24;
  attitudes of whites 26–8; census 5,
  8, 23, 24, 26, 219; desegregation 47,

72–3; emancipation 27;
  hypodescent 8; Japanese 4, 22, 23;
  Jewish people 22, 23, 45; lynchings
  36; melting-pot 43; Mexicans 22,
  132; mixed marriages 7, 21, 22, 24,
  36, 39; mulattos 26, 27, 43, 44;
  octoroon 26, 44; one drop of black
  blood 3, 8, 27, 218; polarisation 7;
  quadroon 26; racial mixing 3, 4, 10,
  43; racism 30; slavery 27; voluntary
  organisations 4

Vanity Fair 19, 26, 27, 31

Washington, Booker T. 44
Wedderburn, Robert 17, 18
Wesley, John 29
West Indians: Afro-Caribbeans *see*
  African Caribbeans; gender
  differences 35–6; mixed marriages
  22, 35–6; population 20; post-war
  immigration 21–2; repatriation 21
West Indies: concubinage 26;
  mulattos 3, 17, 26, 28, 30; racism
  30; slavery 26, 28, 29
Wharton, Arthur 20
Williams, Patricia 71
Wilson, A. 48
working class families: multiracial
  schools 120, 129, 138; observing
  racism 152; racism in school 147,
  160, 230; state schools 120, 129,
  138; survey sample 86, 91

young people: adolescence *see*
  adolescents; black/white culture
  bridged 226–8; dual loyalties 114;
  family relationships 97–8, 101;
  friendships *see* friendships and
  allegiances; marginality 102, 114,
  137, 223–4; marriage preferences
  108, 124–5; most experience of
  racism 158–9
young peoples' identity: black identity
  59, 70, 93–8, 108–10, 222–3; black
  teachers 112–13; centrality of
  identity 110–13; choice of labels
  98–101; definition 220–2; identity
  confusion 105; intermediate
  identity 109, 110; multiracial